I0448075

Healing Hands

The Essential Guide to a Career as a Mental Health Technician

by
Well-Being Publishing

To You,

Thank you!

Table of Contents

Introduction

Welcome to an exploration of a deeply rewarding profession at the heart of modern healthcare—the journey of becoming a Mental Health Technician. As society's understanding and compassion towards mental health continue to evolve, so does the demand for dedicated professionals in this field. The purpose of this book is to shed light on the dynamic role of Mental Health Technicians, diving into the intricacies of the job, and laying out the pathway to a career filled with meaningful interactions and profound impacts on the lives of others.

The landscape of mental health care is changing. It's becoming more integral to the prevailing healthcare system, and with this shift, the role of the Mental Health Technician emerges as an essential piece of the puzzle. This book will help individuals grasp the substantial nature of this role and the importance it holds within the tapestry of patient care. Whether you're a student, contemplating a career change, or seeking insights into mental healthcare professions, this writing aims to be your beacon.

Mental health isn't just about understanding diseases; it's about cultivating a labor of empathy, technical competence, and dedication. As a potential candidate stepping into this field, your journey will demand diligence, a genuine passion for helping others, and a steadfast commitment to personal growth. This introduction seeks to ignite your curiosity, and as you turn each page, allow you to envisage a future within this vital sector.

Let's momentarily consider the world of healthcare. Within this realm, one might envision doctors and nurses in brisk paces down hospital corridors. Yet, beyond this familiar imagery lies a multitude of roles, each with unique contributions that are paramount to the health and wellbeing of patients. The Mental Health Technician stands among these roles, offering specialized assistance that is as intellectually stimulating as it is heart-centered.

In this introductory passage, we look beyond preconceptions and delve into the core of what it means to work as a Mental Health Technician. This is not just a job, but a calling, that invites you to expand your worldview, challenges you to grow personally and professionally, and provides profound fulfillment through service to those in need.

It's imperative to underscore the escalating need for these professionals. As you will learn, the mental health crisis is apparent across the globe, necessitating an armada of passionate individuals ready to step into this space to provide care, to support, to listen, and to be that unwavering pillar for those facing the most challenging times of their lives.

Success as a Mental Health Technician is not merely contingent on the academic knowledge one acquires. Rather, it's the amalgamation of soft skills like empathy and active listening, paired with technical know-how and emotional resilience. This introduction sketches the outline of what these skills look like and how they are instrumental in building a successful career in mental health.

While the heart of this book beats for inspiration, let us not set aside the practicalities. You'll learn about educational pathways, certifications, and nuances of daily responsibilities. Yes, the theory is vital; however, translating that theory into action is where your impact is materialized.

Imagine yourself in the midst of it all; the daily rhythm, the coordination with multidisciplinary teams, and the privileged position of trust you hold. The safeguarding of patient confidentiality, ethical practice, and the perpetual balance of professional boundaries will become clear as you traverse this reading.

Additionally, you will acquaint yourself with the diverse patient populations you will serve. Understanding cultural sensitivities, nuances of various mental disorders, and techniques for building rapport will be laid bare as stepping stones towards effective care.

In this profession, you will often be the frontline in managing crisis situations, a task that requires courage, calm, and an ability to make swift, informed decisions. This introduction will touch upon the gravity of such instances, paving the way for deeper discussions in subsequent chapters.

As you consider the environment you hope to nurture, know that it extends beyond the physical space. A therapeutic environment is also about attitude, approach, and the activities that foster healing. This backdrop is as critical as the clinical tasks at hand, and you will learn to appreciate and craft such a milieu.

Before delving into the nuts and bolts of becoming a Mental Health Technician, we pause to reflect on the human element – the compassion, the reverence for life, and the pure intent that underscores everything in this line of work. Upholding these values is what differentiates a mere job from a true calling.

Embarking on this expedition will also bring to light the critical nature of self-care for those in this profession. The teaching herein is simple yet profound: to give abundantly, one must replenish oneself. This book imparts strategies to ensure you are as attentive to your own wellbeing as you are to your patients'.

Lastly, an eye to the future is keenly focused on throughout these pages. To step into this role is to join a movement, a collective striving for betterment in mental healthcare, driven by innovation, technological advancement, and advocacy. As you stand on the precipice of this ever-expanding field, know your potential contributions could reverberate far and wide.

Allow this introduction to serve as your invitation to discovery, a call to action, and a heartfelt welcome into the fold of mental health professionals. Together, let us embark on this journey of understanding, compassion, and dedication towards a career that promises not just a livelihood, but a life rich with purpose and connection.

Chapter 1:
Understanding Mental Health
and the Role of a Technician

The journey through the landscape of mental health is both a deeply personal and a universal quest, as humanity strives to understand and support those grappling with psychological challenges. In this voyage, the role of a mental health technician emerges as a beacon of practical skill and genuine compassion. As we unfold the map of this rewarding career, we shall explore the intricate tapestry of mental wellbeing, discerning between the ebbs and flows of the human psyche. A mental health technician is the frontline ally in this endeavor, blending technical acuity with an empathetic approach to care that transforms lives. They are the silent guardians, the watchers on the walls of mental restoration, who facilitate healing pathways for those they serve. Each step in this career brims with potential to make an indelible impact on the landscape of healthcare, and it calls to those who seek purpose and passion in their professional lives. By understanding the delicate balance between skill and heart, technicians ready themselves to meet the evolving needs of those in their care, while carving out an essential place for themselves within the pulsating heart of mental health services.

The Evolution of Mental Health Care

The fabric of mental health care has been woven through an intricate and protracted history, often reflective of the broader societal beliefs and scientific understandings of its time. Embarking on this historical journey isn't just about facts; it's a poignant reminder that as future mental health technicians, we are part of a story that is continually unfolding, a narrative shaped by perseverance and evolution. Our role in this domain is informed by a past rich with challenges and triumphs, and it is with this appreciation that we delve into the evolution of mental health care.

The initial understanding of mental illness was heavily shrouded in superstition and fear, often attributed to supernatural forces or divine retribution. Treatment, in ancient times, could involve exorcism or other ritualistic practices believed to rid sufferers of their afflictions. However, the advent of Hippocrates, known as the "Father of Medicine," began to shift the paradigm, as he posited that mental disorders had natural and physical causes. This nascent idea of looking for biological explanations laid the groundwork for future progress.

Move forward to medieval times, and the view of mental illness took a step back into the shadows. The ill were often treated as outcasts or worse, persecuted for their conditions. But these dark times were not to persist. The Renaissance brought about a rebirth of learning and a renewed interest in humanism, sowing the seeds for more compassionate approaches to care.

By the 18th century, significant strides were made with the establishment of some of the first asylums. These institutions aimed to provide care and refuge for individuals with mental health conditions. One pivotal figure during this period was Philippe Pinel, whose advocacy for humane treatment and the unchaining of asylum patients in France marked an enlightened turn in mental healthcare philosophy. Yet, while the intent was to create safe havens, many asylums became overcrowded and fell short of providing truly therapeutic environments.

The 19th century saw further evolution, with pioneers like Dorothea Dix campaigning tirelessly for the establishment of more humane mental health hospitals in the United States. This era heralded the concept that mental illness should be treated medically, not criminally, and paved the way for more reform. However, even as new facilities were built, treatments often remained crude and understudied.

Psychiatry as a professional field began to take shape at the turn of the 20th century. Sigmund Freud's development of psychoanalysis and Carl Jung's analytical psychology provided frameworks for understanding and treating mental distress through talking therapies. The exploration of the human mind through psychology blossomed, further distancing itself from the chains and cells of the past.

The mid-20th century brought dramatic change with the advent of psychopharmacology. The discovery of medications like chlorpromazine, an antipsychotic, offered alternative treatments to the often brutal methods of the past, such as lobotomies and electroconvulsive therapy. Psychiatric medication created a revolution in care, allowing many individuals to live more fully outside of institutional walls.

However, the large-scale closure of psychiatric hospitals, a movement known as deinstitutionalization, beginning in the 1960s, had complex repercussions. While it aimed to empower individuals through community-based care, it also led to gaps in services and a rise in homelessness and incarceration among the mentally ill who did not receive adequate support.

The late 20th century and early 21st century are characterized by an unprecedented growth in our understanding of mental health disorders. Neuroimaging and advances in genetics have provided insights into the biological underpinnings of many conditions, reshaping diagnostic and treatment approaches. Additionally, the recognition of the importance of psychotherapy has evolved, with evidence-based therapies such as cognitive-behavioral therapy becoming standard practice.

Today's mental health care is a far cry from its rudimentary beginnings. Integration of care, where mental health services are combined with general health services, and telehealth, providing remote access to mental health professionals, epitomize the modern, connected approach. Mental health has finally begun to achieve parity with physical health in many healthcare systems, though there remains much to achieve.

As future mental health technicians, we must recognize our role in this still-changing landscape. We bear the responsibility to provide empathetic, knowledgeable, and up-to-date care that reflects the lessons learned through history. Our work will contribute to further innovations in treatment, understanding, and the de-stigmatization of mental illness.

Each stride made in mental health care, from early herbal remedies to the latest digital therapy apps, is a testament to human resilience and innovation. It's also a stark reminder of our responsibility to continue pushing the boundaries of what we know, to listen intently to the lived experiences of those we help, and to be compassionate facilitators in their journey towards holistic well-being.

The historical arc of mental health care tells a story of a field defined by continuous reinvention, a trait that is instrumental in understanding and embracing the work ahead. Mental health technicians become part of this storied history, carrying the torch forward, upholding the dignity of patients, and ensuring care evolves in both compassionate and scientifically sound ways.

To those stepping into the field, you are joining a lineage of care providers who have paved the path to the present. And as you venture into this work, let this history empower you. You stand on the shoulders of giants and become part of the tapestry that will form the future of mental health care—a future where everyone's mental health is respected, prioritized, and expertly supported.

Defining the Mental Health Technician

As we delve into the core of what it means to be a mental health technician (MHT), it's essential to crystallize our understanding of this pivotal role. An MHT serves as a cornerstone in the broader mental healthcare ecosystem, aiding individuals grappling with a multitude of mental health challenges. They stand as allies, caretakers, and crucial frontline workers in both inpatient and outpatient settings.

Mental health technicians are the unsung heroes in the trenches of clinical environments, extending both technical support and compassionate care. They navigate the complex waters of patients' emotional and behavioral conditions, employing a keen sense of empathy and understanding that cannot be overstated. The true essence of an MHT lies in their ability to juggle a profound assortment of duties with a poised and patient-centric approach.

But what exactly are these duties? The breadth of responsibilities encompassed in the MHT's role is expansive. They conduct routine patient observations, contribute to treatment planning, and assist with therapeutic interventions. It's their versatile skillset that often makes the most visible impact on a patient's day-to-day experience within a care setting.

At the heart of the mental health technician's role is the patient. MHTs support patients' basic needs, from hygiene assistance to nutritional guidance, while also ensuring that psychological and therapeutic needs are addressed. This supportive care is pivotal in reinforcing the treatment and recovery process, essentially making MHTs integral in fostering patient progress.

From monitoring vitals to meticulously documenting patients' behaviors and responses to treatments, MHTs play an active role in the care team. Data provided by technicians often guide treatment adjustments, and their observations can yield invaluable insights into a patient's mental state – insights that even the most seasoned psychiatrist may not discern without them.

One might wonder about the skill set required to excel as a mental health technician. Beyond the foundational medical knowledge surrounding mental health conditions, MHTs must possess exceptional communication skills. They often serve as the conduit between mental health professionals and patients, necessitating clear and effective dialogue among all parties involved.

Similarly essential is an MHT's ability to remain calm and collected in potentially volatile situations. Crises do arise within mental health facilities, and it's during these moments that MHTs demonstrate their crucial role in maintaining a safe environment for everyone. Their training allows them to effectively de-escalate conflicts and manage emergency situations with both precision and empathy.

The nurturing nature of the MHT is not to be overlooked; it stems from a deep-seated passion for helping others and a genuine desire to contribute positively to patients' lives. Mental health technicians often form strong therapeutic relationships with those in their care, serving as a beacon of stability and trust.

Interpersonal skills are also central to the work of an MHT. They often navigate diverse cultural landscapes, requiring sensitivity and adaptability to a wide range of patient backgrounds. Cultural competence is not just an asset but a necessity in this field to deliver inclusive and respectful care.

For those considering a career as a mental health technician, it's important to understand the investment in personal growth and learning that the role demands. It's a pathway defined by continuous evolution – as treatment modalities shift, so must the techniques and approaches employed by MHTs. The commitment to ongoing education and adaptability is at the forefront of excellence in this field.

Amidst the many roles in mental healthcare, the mental health technician is uniquely positioned to impact individuals' lives significantly. Think of the MHT as the backbone of daily operations within mental health facilities, combining technical knowledge with heartfelt empathy to create a supportive and healing atmosphere.

Let's not forget, the robustness of an MHT's role is mirrored by the challenges that accompany it. The emotional toll of working in mental health can be substantial; thus, an effective MHT equips themselves with a toolbox of self-care practices. Acknowledging the weight of what they carry for others is key to sustaining their well-being and continued ability to serve.

Ultimately, defining a mental health technician cannot be distilled to a mere job description. It's a vocation, a calling that beckons those resilient and dedicated individuals who seek to play an active role in the healing journey of others. It demands a symbiosis of skill and spirit that characterizes the finest in healthcare professions.

If you find within you a wellspring of empathy, a steady hand for the tumultuous seas of mental health, and a relentless drive to learn and grow, the path of the mental health technician may very well be your calling. It's a challenging yet immeasurably rewarding pursuit that beckons aspirants to step forward and make a tangible difference in the realm of mental health care.

In the chapters to come, we will further explore the terrain that mental health technicians navigate, illuminating the demands and rewards of this essential role. With each passing section, you'll gain deeper insight, not only into the responsibilities and required competencies of an MHT but also into the profound impact one can make in this dynamic field of care.

Chapter 2:
The Growing Demand for
Mental Health Technicians

In the wake of recognizing the sheer magnitude of mental health challenges facing society today, it's clear that Mental Health Technicians (MHTs) are more crucial than ever before. As we venture further into a world where the prominence of mental wellbeing can't be understated, MHTs emerge as indispensable support systems within the healthcare matrix. The demand for these skilled professionals is surging, propelled by a societal awakening to the mental health crisis and its ripple effects across communities. With an empathetic touch and a keen understanding of psychological care, MHTs provide a scaffold for individuals grappling with their mental health, filling a gap that has been long felt in healthcare services. Job market trends reflect this growth, showing a trajectory that promises diversity, opportunity, and the chance to make a tangible difference. For those with a spark to serve and a drive to thrive in a role that truly matters, the path of an MHT offers a beacon of hope and fulfillment. In this chapter, we unfurl the tapestry of the expanding need for MHTs and the vitality of their role—illuminating the way forward for aspirants ready to step into a career where passion and purpose converge.

Mental Health Crisis and the Need for Supportive Care

As we venture deeper into the world of mental health care, we acknowledge a landscape where the demand for professionals is growing by the day. The mental health crisis is not an isolated phenomenon; it is a global challenge affecting millions. Each individual battling mental health issues carries a unique story, and behind each story lies the need for compassionate, supportive care.

The term crisis might evoke images of dramatic events; however, in the realm of mental health, a crisis can be any situation where an individual's behavior poses a threat to their well-being or that of others. At the heart of this is a cry for help, an urgent call for professionals who can bridge the gap between suffering and healing. Mental health technicians stand on the frontline of this battle, serving as an indispensable part of the support network.

The rise in mental health conditions such as anxiety, depression, and substance abuse has led to an unprecedented strain on mental health services. It paints a clear picture: there's a profound need for mental health technicians who can provide ongoing, supportive care. This supportive care isn't just about managing symptoms; it's about fostering an environment where recovery can flourish.

Supportive care extends beyond the walls of therapy rooms and hospitals. It is present in schools, homes, and communities. It is in the gentle, yet skilled hands of mental health technicians, who offer day-to-day interactions that can be as impactful as any medication or therapy session. These technicians provide a continuity of care that is essential for many patients' long-term recovery and well-being.

This role in supportive care is not a passive one. It requires active engagement, genuine empathy, and a deep understanding of the complexities of mental health. Mental health technicians are taught to listen, not just to the words being said but also to the silent messages conveyed through behavior and emotion. This level of attunement can make all the difference to someone feeling seen and heard.

Let's not mistake supportive care for a lower level of care. It is a specialized, skill-intensive service that mental health technicians provide. Their work is rooted in evidence-based practices and the latest in psychological research, ensuring that their support is both empathetic and effective. Their interactions can build trust that encourages patients to engage more fully in their treatment plans.

The reality is that many mental health conditions cannot be treated in a vacuum. They require a multi-faceted approach, where medication might be coupled with psychotherapy and consistent support. Mental health technicians are instrumental in carrying out this comprehensive care, often being the ones to maintain the continuity that is vital for patients navigating the complexities of their conditions.

As the prevalence of mental illness grows, so does the societal recognition that mental health is just as important as physical health. This awareness has led to increased funding, legislation, and programs dedicated to improving mental health care systems. Mental health technicians play a crucial role in implementing these advancements and ensuring that they reach those in need.

The need for supportive care also emphasizes the importance of early intervention. The presence of mental health technicians in various settings enables quicker identification of mental health concerns, and in turn, attempts to address them before they escalate. It's this proactive stance that can prevent crises and profoundly change the trajectory of a person's life.

The work of mental health technicians is not without its challenges. It requires resilience, patience, and unwavering dedication. But it is also work that illuminates the human soul, that uncovers the strength and resilience that lie within the fabric of our shared humanity. It's a calling that answers not just to the needs of individuals, but to the needs of a society grappling with a mental health crisis.

Through the effective provision of supportive care, mental health technicians help to alleviate the burden on overtaxed mental health professionals, such as psychiatrists and psychologists. They are the additional hands and hearts that are desperately needed in the high-pressure environment of mental health care.

What's more, the role of supportive care is ever-evolving. As our society becomes more complex, the challenges to mental health also transform, demanding adaptable, trained professionals who are capable of evolving alongside them. Mental health technicians are at the forefront, meeting this challenge with both proficiency and compassion.

In this era of ever-increasing mental health needs, the supportive care provided by mental health technicians has never been more vital. They are the embodiment of the saying "to care is to act." Their everyday actions speak volumes about their commitment to those they serve and to a brighter future for mental health care.

Indeed, the journey of a mental health technician is marked with challenges, but also with immeasurable rewards. By becoming trained in this field, you're not just pursuing a career; you're embracing a mission to assist individuals in their darkest hours, and in doing so, you bring more light into the world. The need for supportive care is clear, and the call for dedicated mental health technicians is loud and resounding.

Employment Outlook and Job Market Trends

As we delve into the realities of the modern mental health landscape, it is crucial to understand the trajectory that job market trends and employment outlooks are taking, particularly for those interested in the role of a mental health technician. This profession, essential in the matrix of mental health services, is experiencing a notable surge in demand. The reasons behind this growth are multifaceted, stemming from a heightened awareness of mental health issues, societal changes, and an evolution in how care is provided.

The Bureau of Labor Statistics (BLS) projects that the employment of mental health technicians, also known as psychiatric technicians, is expected to grow faster than the average for all occupations over the next decade. This expansion is driven, in part, by an aging population, which will require an increase in mental health services, as well as the ongoing destigmatization of mental health care which encourages more individuals to seek help.

Another contributor to this trend is the integration of mental health services into general healthcare services. As hospitals and primary care settings increasingly recognize the importance of mental health in overall wellness, the demand for trained professionals to provide these services at the first point of contact continues to rise.

The job market for mental health technicians is undergoing a diversification process. Historically, these professionals have been employed predominantly in psychiatric hospitals and residential mental health facilities. Today, we see an expansion with opportunities in outpatient care centers, correctional facilities, community health centers, schools, and even corporate environments that are bolstering wellness programs.

Technological advancements are also reshaping the field. The rise of telepsychiatry and mobile health apps for mental wellness mean that technicians need to be proficient with new tools and means of delivery. This requires a continuous learning approach to keep up with the digitalization of mental health services, opening up remote work opportunities and expanding the reach of those needing care.

Regionally, certain areas are witnessing a more pronounced demand due to varying factors such as population density, prevalence of mental health conditions, and availability of services. For those willing to relocate, this can present a wealth of opportunities. Practitioners may find a dynamic job market in urban areas, while rural regions offer the chance to fill gaps in service and make a significant community impact.

Alongside these positive trends, it's important to note the challenges that influence the job market. Insurance coverage and mental health parity laws affect service accessibility and staffing needs. Economic fluctuations can also impact government funding for public mental health services, which in turn affects employment opportunities. Mental health technicians must be adaptable and prepared to navigate these hurdles with resilience and resourcefulness.

The current societal focus on mental health and well-being is creating a favorable professional climate. Employers are seeking individuals who not only have the technical skills necessary for the job but who also exhibit a passion for helping others, emotional intelligence, and the adaptability required to thrive in diverse settings.

Furthermore, the mental health technician profession serves as a stepping stone for many in the field of mental health. This role provides invaluable experience that can pave the way to advanced positions. Career growth into supervisory roles, specializations in certain types of care, or progress into other roles such as licensed counselors or social workers can all stem from the foundational role of the mental health technician.

The consolidation of integrated care models, where physical and mental health are treated in tandem, has prompted an interdisciplinary approach to recruitment. Mental health technicians are increasingly working alongside a broad spectrum of healthcare professionals, which means that their exposure and learning potential within the job market have significantly broadened.

In response to these factors, educational institutions are tailoring programs to meet the growing need for mental health technicians. This is reflected in an increase in relevant degree programs, certifications, and training opportunities aimed at equipping prospective technicians with both the knowledge and practical skills necessary to excel in the field.

The COVID-19 pandemic has also had a lasting impact on the job market. The resulting isolation, anxiety, and other psychological stresses have underscored the essential nature of mental health services. This has, in turn, catalyzed additional funding and an increase in job openings for mental health professionals, including technicians, to address the surge in mental health needs.

Ultimately, the employment outlook and job market trends for mental health technicians are not only strong but also evolving. For those passionate about making a difference, the field offers a broad and ever-expanding canvas to apply their skills and compassion. It's an opportunity to be at the forefront of societal change, playing a vital role in improving the mental well-being of individuals and communities alike.

Remember, each step taken in this career is a step towards progress, both for the individual and for the larger goal of providing accessible, high-quality mental health care. As the job market continues to thrive, so does the opportunity for mental health technicians to grow, innovate, and contribute to a healthier, more supportive society.

Chapter 3:
Essential Skills and Qualities for Success

Success in the mental health field isn't just a matter of education and experience; it's equally about the personal qualities you bring to the table. In Chapter 3, we delve into the essential skills and qualities that forge a successful Mental Health Technician. Possessing strong interpersonal and communication abilities isn't just desirable—it's imperative. You'll learn how the power of empathy and the ability to actively listen create a foundation for effective patient support. We'll dissect the technical know-how and hands-on capabilities that are crucial for delivering top-notch care. But it doesn't end there; we'll also uncover the immense value of emotional resilience. Balancing compassion with self-care, maintaining your equilibrium amidst challenging situations—these are the hallmarks of a technician who doesn't merely survive in this field but thrives. With these insights, you'll be equipped to embody the excellence that sets apart those who succeed in making a real difference in the lives of those struggling with mental health challenges.

Interpersonal and Communication Skills

At the core of a Mental Health Technician's daily work lies the profound ability to connect and communicate with patients, colleagues, and industry professionals. The mastery of interpersonal and communication skills isn't just a nicety; it's an absolute necessity for those who choose to serve in this calling. Empathy and active listening form the bedrock of such skills, allowing technicians to listen to patients without preconceived judgments, therapeutically engage, and foster a sense of trust and safety that is indispensable in mental health care.

Effective communication extends beyond mere words. It's an art that balances speaking and silence, questioning and understanding, directness and discretion. For a Mental Health Technician, verbal skills must be tailored to meet the varied needs of patients whose ability to process information can be vastly different. Crafting messages that are clear, concise, and compassionate can significantly influence a patient's responsiveness and progress. But remember, it's not just what you say, it's also how you say it.

Nonverbal cues are equally potent. Your posture, gestures, and facial expressions can speak volumes, often louder than your spoken words. These subtle signals can reinforce trust and rapport, or they can undo it. Great care must be taken to ensure that your nonverbal communication aligns with your spoken intent, nurturing a harmonious environment conducive to healing.

Beyond one-on-one interactions, documentation and written communication skills are integral to a Mental Health Technician's role. The clarity in your notes, reports, and patient files can significantly aid in the continuity of care, ensuring all team members are informed and aligned. Crafting succinct yet detailed notes is a skill that, when honed, transforms into a powerful tool for patient advocacy and team collaboration.

Feedback loops are another cornerstone of effective communication, especially within interdisciplinary teams. The ability to give and receive constructive feedback empowers continuous improvement and personal growth. It allows teams to adjust treatment plans, refine approaches, and strengthen relationships, ultimately elevating the quality of care provided.

The capacity to manage conflicts is a testament to a technician's interpersonal adeptness. The mental health field, like any other, is not immune to disagreements and tensions. However, a technician's ability to navigate these situations with tact, diplomacy, and a conflict-resolution mindset can mitigates stress and fosters a supportive environment for both colleagues and patients.

Cultural competency is more than just a buzzword; it's a critical component of communication. The ability to interact effectively with individuals from diverse backgrounds is not just about respect; it's about providing individualized care that honors the patient's cultural, social, and personal values. Being culturally aware and sensitive amplifies your capability to connect and be effective in your role.

Empowerment through communication is a transformative technique that Mental Health Technicians can integrate into their practice. Encouraging patients to articulate their thoughts and feelings, validating their experiences, and reinforcing their autonomy and decision-making skills, underpin an ethos of respect and collaboration that can profoundly accelerate recovery.

Teaching and education, too, are part of a Mental Health Technician's repertoire of communication skills. Whether instructing a patient on coping strategies, guiding them through therapeutic exercises, or providing insight into medication management, the ability to break down complex concepts into digestible, actionable steps is invaluable.

With the influx of technology, electronic communication now plays a pivotal role. Email etiquette, electronic health record (EHR) proficiency, and savvy in utilizing telehealth platforms are now part of the fundamental communication skill set for today's Mental Health Technicians. These skills enable efficient and effective exchanges that respect privacy and enhance care.

Understanding and respecting boundaries is essential in nurturing therapeutic relationships. Effective communication involves recognizing and maintaining professional limits, ensuring a clear delineation between patient and caregiver roles. This leads to a stronger, healthier therapeutic relationship and better outcomes.

Conflict management also includes de-escalation techniques, an area where communication prowess is crucial. As a Mental Health Technician, you may encounter challenging behaviors or crisis situations. Reacting calmly, speaking soothingly, and utilizing evidence-based de-escalation strategies can quickly diffuse tension and prevent escalation.

The importance of teamwork cannot be overstated, and the linchpin of any successful team is communication. As a Mental Health Technician, you'll often work within a multidisciplinary team, each member relying on timely and clear communication to perform their role effectively. The contribution of clear articulation of observations and insights ensures the team's synergy and the patient's well-being.

Crisis communication is a specialized subset of these skills. In unpredicted, high-stress situations, conveying critical information with clarity and speed can be life-saving. These scenarios demand situational awareness, a calm demeanor, and precision in instructions and information sharing.

Lastly, while these interpersonal and communication skills are nuanced and dimensional, they are also teachable and learnable. Continual learning and practice can refine these skills over time, shaping you into not just a Mental Health Technician but a communication virtuoso. Your dedication to mastering these skills can ripple through your career, lifting your capabilities and the care you provide to new heights.

Technical Knowledge and Hands-On Abilities

This is a core aspect of a mental health technician's prowess, bridging the gap between theoretical understanding and actionable skills in the robust ecosystem of mental health care. As we explore this crucial sub-section, envision embarking on a journey to master a toolkit that can transform lives. Possessing a strong foundation in technical knowledge and hands-on capabilities is essential to delivering effective care and supporting the multidisciplinary teams that define modern mental health practices.

The technical knowledge for a mental health technician is not limited to a single facet; it encompasses a gamut of psychiatric conditions, treatment plans, and an intricate understanding of human behavior. To be effective in this role, one must endeavor to comprehend the nuances of mental illnesses — not purely from a clinical perspective but also from a holistic viewpoint that considers the patient's full circle of life.

Hands-on abilities are quintessential in this realm. For instance, knowing how to accurately monitor vital signs or administer medications aren't mere tasks—they're lifelines. These skills require precision, dexterity, and an unwavering commitment to patient safety. You'll find that these hands-on interactions, while often brief, have lasting impacts on the therapeutic relationship.

Effective communication, too, is a cornerstone of technical capability. It's not enough to speak; one must converse in a way that educates, informs, and provides comfort. You'll learn to document patient behaviors meticulously, ensuring that narratives are clear and concise for fellow caregivers, thus fostering a seamless continuum of care.

Safety procedures form another critical segment of your hands-on learning. In mental health facilities, there's a pervasive need to be vigilant in recognizing potential crises before they escalate. A mental health technician must not only anticipate such events but be adept at employing non-violent crisis intervention techniques to defuse tension and maintain an environment conducive to healing.

Operating within therapeutic boundaries requires deft maneuvers between being a source of support and maintaining professional conduct. Here lies a delicate balancing act, where you provide compassionate care without overstepping the boundaries that keep you and your patients safe. This balance demands a certain finesse that you'll cultivate through experience and reflective practice.

In an age where digital technology increasingly interfaces with healthcare, a mental health technician's technical acumen also extends to electronic health records (EHRs). Mastery of EHR systems is non-negotiable as these digital tools are pivotal for efficient and effective patient care management.

Observational skills are another non-negotiable. The subtleties of a patient's non-verbal cues often speak volumes about their internal state. You'll learn to trust your perception, to observe the minute changes in behavior that may indicate progress or concern. It's these insights, drawn from attentive observation, that can guide interventions and enhance patient outcomes.

Therapeutic engagement tactics also form part of the hands-on abilities. Whether it's leading a group therapy session or utilizing recreational therapy to promote mental well-being, the application of these methods demands a deep understanding of group dynamics and individual comfort levels.

When intervening in acute situations, your heart may race, adrenaline may surge, but your training enables you to act with precision and calm—administering first aid, supporting a patient undergoing a panic attack, or swiftly implementing suicide prevention protocols.

Staying abreast of emerging trends and technologies in mental healthcare is a perpetual commitment. It's essential to be well-versed in new treatments, especially as our understanding of mental health evolves. Your willingness to learn and adapt is as crucial as the foundational knowledge you build upon.

Simulations and role-play exercises often serve as the training grounds for refining hands-on skills. Immersing yourself in these simulations, you'll gain confidence and the ability to react purposefully and compassionately in a range of scenarios.

Maintaining patient dignity during personal care tasks not only requires technical skill but a respectful approach. You become a guardian of dignity, ensuring that each action, from assisting with personal hygiene to providing mobility support, is carried out with the utmost respect for the person in your care.

No aspect of a mental health technician's job should be underestimated—each nuance, each learned reaction, and each applied piece of knowledge forms the mosaic of your career. The blend of technical expertise and hands-on practice is a dance between science and art; it's where compassion meets capability, where theory encounters practice, and where you, as a future mental health technician, will make an indelible impact on the lives of those you serve.

Remember, mastery doesn't occur overnight. It's achieved through consistency, a quest for knowledge, and an unwavering dedication to the craft of mental health care. As you continue on this path, your skill set will grow, and your capacity to change lives—for that is the true measure of success in this profession—will expand beyond measure. Embrace this journey with an open heart and a keen mind, and the rewards of your labor will be as profound as the lives you touch.

Emotional Resilience and Self-Care

As we delve into the essential skills and qualities necessary for a successful career as a Mental Health Technician, we encounter a vital, yet often underrated component: emotional resilience and self-care. The ability to maintain one's own emotional stability in the face of adversity is not just a personal asset; it's a professional requirement in mental health care. Much like an athlete who conditions their body for a race, Mental Health Technicians must cultivate their emotional resilience to navigate the ups and downs of their work with strength and grace.

Mental health work is inherently challenging. As a technician, you will be exposed to a wide array of human experiences, many of which may be fraught with pain, crisis, and emotional turmoil. Your capacity to remain composed and offer support hinges on your emotional resilience. This quality enables you to recover quickly from the inevitable setbacks and difficult interactions that are part of the job.

Crafting emotional resilience is akin to building a fortress within oneself. It involves recognizing your emotional triggers and developing strategies to cope with them effectively. It might mean taking a moment to breathe deeply when you feel overwhelmed or learning to decompress after a long day through activities that nourish your spirit.

Resilience also benefits from a mindset of growth and adaptability. Embrace the lessons each challenge teaches you. Reflect after difficult encounters and consider what skills or tools might better equip you for next time. Sometimes resilience is about bending rather than breaking—and then learning to straighten back up, fortified from the experience.

Self-care is the twin pillar that supports emotional resilience. It's a practice that's often preached but just as often overlooked in its importance. As someone entering the mental health field, you must prioritize your mental and physical well-being. You cannot pour from an empty cup, and in the demanding environment of mental health care, where burnout is real, regular self-care is not an indulgence—it's an imperative.

Self-care manifests in various forms and is highly individual. For some, it's physical activity that keeps the mind clear; for others, it might be quiet time with a book or engaging in creative pursuits. Social connections can also be part of self-care, providing laughter, compassion, and understanding outside of the professional milieu.

Importantly, self-care includes setting boundaries. As you support others in navigating their emotional landscapes, it's critical to know your own limits. Learn to say no, to delegate, and to recognize when you need to step back. Protecting your time and emotional energy is not selfish—it's necessary for sustainability in this field.

Moreover, developing a self-care routine should be an ongoing process. Just as an athlete doesn't train for a marathon in a single session, you shouldn't expect to master self-care overnight. Embed rituals into your day that help you unplug from work and recharge your batteries. This routine could include meditation, journaling, or spending time in nature—anything that helps you maintain balance.

One aspect of self-care that is sometimes neglected is professional support. Do not underestimate the value of therapy or supervision for yourself. Having a space to unpack the vicissitudes of your work can be incredibly beneficial. It's not just patients who need to talk through their experiences; Mental Health Technicians also require a sounding board to process their feelings and prevent compassion fatigue.

Education about the concept of vicarious trauma and strategies to mitigate its effects should be a priority. Just as you will learn how to support others, it is critical that you learn techniques to shield yourself from becoming secondary victims of the trauma you witness. Recognizing the signs of vicarious trauma in yourself and peers is key to fostering a supportive community within your workplace where everyone watches out for each other.

Remember, emotional resilience and self-care are not static; they're practices that develop and evolve over time. As you learn from each experience in your professional journey, your toolkit for maintaining emotional health will expand. Reflect regularly on your self-care practices, adjusting them as necessary to ensure they remain effective and congruent with your evolving needs.

It's also worth noting that the culture of the workplace can greatly influence your resilience. Seek out environments that value the well-being of their staff, where senior professionals lead by example in self-care and encourage their teams to take well-being seriously. In such environments, you'll find that emotional resilience is not only supported but celebrated.

Lastly, never underestimate the power of community. Connection with colleagues who understand the unique pressures of the mental health field can be incredibly enriching. These relationships can serve as a vital network of support, validation, and shared wisdom. Together, you can navigate the challenges and celebrate the triumphs that come with the meaningful work of a Mental Health Technician.

In conclusion, emotional resilience and self-care are not just supplementary skills but core components of a sustainable and satisfying career in mental health care. As you prepare to enter this field, recognize that the care you provide to yourself is just as crucial as the care you offer to others. Your ability to remain resilient and well will not only impact your longevity in the profession but also the quality of care you're able to provide. Cultivate these aspects with the same dedication you apply to learning technical skills and knowledge, and watch as they become the bedrock of your professional and personal fulfillment.

Chapter 4:
Educational Pathways and Certifications

As we sail further into the ocean of mental health knowledge, Chapter 4 serves as a compass for navigating through the various educational routes and certifications necessary for a career as a Mental Health Technician. Embark on a journey that begins with understanding the foundational degree programs and courses that will imbue you with the knowledge and skills essential for this rewarding profession. Uncover the significance of targeted certification and licensure, key milestones that authenticate your expertise and dedication to the field. Moreover, recognize the value of continuing education and specialized training, essential for keeping your practices current and your passion ignited. These educational pathways aren't simply a series of checkboxes but stepping-stones to building a profound and impactful career, shaping your ability to touch the lives of those grappling with mental health challenges and contributing to the broader canvas of healthcare innovation.

Degree Programs and Courses

As we transition from earlier discussions regarding the role, demand, and essential attributes of a mental health technician, it becomes crucial to focus on the educational pathways that pave the way forward. Just as sculptors require chisels to craft art, mental health technicians need education and training to cultivate their expertise. Numerous institutions offer degree programs and courses that align with the calling of this profession. In this context, we delve into the avenues that can enrich your professional journey, tailor your skill set, and enhance your capability to make a meaningful impact in the lives of individuals seeking mental health support.

The pathway to becoming a distinguished mental health technician often begins with pursuing relevant educational qualifications. Many colleges and universities offer associate degree programs in mental health technology or psychiatric technology, providing a solid foundation in the field. These two-year programs blend coursework in psychology, biology, and counseling with practical clinical experiences, giving students exposure to a range of mental health care settings.

For individuals seeking to delve deeper and further distinguish themselves, bachelor's degree programs in psychology, social work, or a related field can be a gateway to more advanced positions within mental health care. These four-year programs expand on the complexities of human behavior, research methods, and therapeutic techniques. Accrued knowledge from bachelor's programs enables graduates to navigate the rich tapestry of mental health care with an even greater understanding and adaptability.

It is essential, regardless of the degree level, to seek out courses that cover a spectrum of relevant topics. Core subjects often include crisis intervention, substance abuse, group therapy dynamics, psychiatric terminology, and behavioral science. Additional classes may offer specialized training in areas such as gerontology, child and adolescent mental health, or developmental disabilities, allowing for fine-tuned expertise in subfields of interest.

Indeed, real-world practice is where your knowledge will be pressed into service, and thus, clinical rotations or internships are often integrated into degree programs. Such experiences can be pivotal, affording students the opportunity to witness the application of theories in practice, to engage directly with patients, and to navigate the nuances of regulated environments under the tutelage of seasoned professionals.

As mental health awareness grows, so too does the recognition of specialized disciplines within the field. Programs that offer courses in PTSD, trauma-informed care, or addiction provide critical skills for those destined to work with specific populations. Being well-versed in these areas will not only enhance your ability to provide exceptional care but also fortify your value as a professional in the eyes of employers.

For those impassioned by the convergence of technology and mental health, courses focusing on telehealth, electronic health records, and health informatics are increasingly prevalent. Mastery of such technologies is becoming indispensable, as the digital transformation of healthcare services renders them vital components of contemporary practice.

Advanced degree options such as master's programs in clinical psychology, counseling, or psychiatric nursing build upon foundational education and open the door to supervisory or more specialized roles within the mental health field. Remember, with every additional certification, degree, or course, you expand not only your skill set but also the breadth of impact you can have on the emotional and psychological welfare of those in need.

Yet, it should be understood that there is no single ordained path to becoming a mental health technician. The essence of education in this field is not merely the accumulation of knowledge but the personal transformation it engenders within you. This enlightenment empowers you to carry out your duties with compassion, professional acumen, and a commitment to human dignity.

Should you feel uncertain about which educational route to undertake, consult academic advisors or professionals already working in the field. They can provide insight into which degree programs and courses helped shape their careers and assist you in charting a course that resonates with your aspirations and the demands of the workforce.

Extracurricular activities and workshops, too, can complement formal education. These avenues offer additional resources and networking opportunities, which are paramount in the interconnected world of mental health care. They also reflect your proactive stance toward enhancing your expertise and passion for aiding those with mental health challenges.

Financial considerations are, without doubt, a reality when pursuing higher education. However, remember that an investment in your education is an investment in the lives you will touch as a mental health technician. Scholarships, grants, and loan forgiveness programs for those entering health service fields can ease this burden and should be explored with due diligence.

As we wind down this exploration of degree programs and courses, let it be reaffirmed: education is both the root and the route of professional competency. Whether you're at the outset of your educational journey or looking to ascend to new heights of expertise, your pursuit of knowledge is commendable. It is the fertile ground from which your ability to serve as a beacon of hope and healing in mental health care will grow.

Remember, while the demands of academia can be rigorous, the rewards mirror the effort invested. Visualize the day when you apply your learning to better someone's mental health – that transformative moment is worth every hour of study, every exam, every practical lesson learned.

In the next section, we will delve into the realms of certification and licensure requirements, which are the credentials that will officially endorse you as a trusted mental health professional. Your educational foundation will be your stepping stone into this next critical phase of your career development.

Certification and Licensure Requirements

As we pivot from understanding the educational background required to flourish as a Mental Health Technician, it's crucial to discuss certification and licensure. The labyrinth of certification and licensure in the mental health field is a vital piece of the puzzle for those aspiring to make a difference in the lives of individuals grappling with mental health issues. Ensuring that you are not only qualified but also authorized to practice is the linchpin to a legitimate and impactful career.

The specifics of certification and licensure vary tremendously across different regions. Typically, to be recognized as a certified Mental Health Technician (MHT), you must satisfy certain criteria set by recognized accrediting bodies. Often, this includes completing an accredited training program, which may culminate in a certificate, diploma, or degree, depending on the level of complexity and depth of the program.

Once the educational mandates are completed, the next stride is to pass a certification exam. This examination is designed to gauge your grasp of the requisite knowledge and skills essential to perform effectively in the role. Organizations like the American Association of Psychiatric Technicians (AAPT) confer certifications at varying levels, ranging from basic to advanced, tailored to match the depth of education and hands-on experience attained.

Certification is more than a formal credential; it is an adamant statement of professional prowess. It validates your commitment to the field and your determination to provide the best care possible. Employers value these certifications, often seeing them as a measure of competence and professionalism. Holding a certification can give you an edge in the competitive job market and sometimes, it may even be a hiring prerequisite.

However, one must be acutely aware that certification is not a one-time affair. It demands ongoing education and renewal periodically to ensure you remain on the cutting-edge of best practices and emerging knowledge in mental health care.

Licensure plays a different but equally critical role. While not all US states require MHTs to be licensed, there are a few that do. Licensure usually involves meeting educational standards, obtaining a specified amount of supervised clinical experience, and passing a state-specific exam. It's imperative to check with your state's health board to understand your state's specific requirements, as they can vary substantively.

In licensed states, it's illegal to practice without this credential, and operating without it can lead to severe repercussions. It's also worth noting that licensure can open doors to other career advancement opportunities, such as supervisory roles or more specialized positions within the mental health field.

Both certification and licensure not only underscore your qualifications but also serve as a guarantee to your patients and their families that you are competent and trustworthy. They're a testament to your fortitude as an MHT and can be incredibly fulfilling milestones on your professional journey.

Maintaining certification and licensure also typically requires continuing education units (CEUs). These educational activities keep you at the forefront of evolving trends, new treatments, and emerging research. They represent a commitment to lifelong learning and an investment in your professional expertise.

Pursuing additional certifications or specializations can also be a magnificent way to distinguish yourself. For instance, certifications in areas like substance abuse counseling or geriatric care can open new doors and elevate the breadth of your expertise and value as an MHT.

It's essential to stay organized and aware of renewal periods for your certification and licensure. Letting these credentials lapse can lead to a halt in your ability to practice and could damage your professional reputation. Thus, keeping track of your credentialing through proper documentation and timely renewal is as important as obtaining them in the first place.

Remember, becoming a Mental Health Technician is not just about acquiring knowledge; it's about embodying a set of values dedicated to improving mental health and fostering a trustworthy environment for those in need. Certification and licensure are the gateways to manifesting those values into a tangible, valuable, and legal service.

In the dynamic world of mental health care, your commitment to acquiring certification and licensure is an ongoing testament to your dedication to bettering lives. As you journey through this process, embrace the challenge with open arms—it's a crucial step toward fulfilling your calling to make a meaningful difference in the world of mental health.

While the journey to certification and licensure may seem daunting, it's an empowering process that strengthens not only your professional credibility but also reinforces your personal growth and resilience. Each step of certification and licensure is a step toward gaining respect and acknowledgment in your chosen field, but more importantly, it's a stride toward potential transformation in the lives of those who struggle.

To conclude, while the certification and licensure requirements in the field of Mental Health Technicians can pose challenges, they are foundational stones in building a career based on proficiency, integrity, and conscientious care. These processes instill confidence in your patients, reassure your employer about the quality of your practice, and assure the public about the standards of mental healthcare provision. Understanding and meeting these requirements are your key to a successful and rewarding career that can truly impact lives and help strengthen our communities.

Continuing Education and Specializations

If there's a cornerstone in the career of a Mental Health Technician (MHT), it's the commitment to lifelong learning and self-improvement. As you've discovered in the previous chapters, the landscape of mental health demands a robust foundation of knowledge and skills. But what differentiates a good technician from a great one? The passion to dive deeper, to not only understand the broader concepts but to also specialize and refine your expertise. Continuing education and specialization are not just buzzwords; they represent a path to expertise that can lead to better patient outcomes, more fulfilling work, and a wealthier career in every sense of the term.

Continuing education comes in many forms, from advanced degrees to specialized certifications. It's an investment in your future that can propel your career forward, allowing you to specialize in areas such as substance abuse, geriatric care, pediatric mental health, or forensics. Education sharpens your skills, broadens your knowledge, and makes you a more valuable team member in any mental health setting.

Gone are the days when an initial certification or degree was enough. The field of mental health is dynamic, with research constantly pushing the boundaries of what we know. It is vital that as an MHT, you stay abreast of these changes. Not only will this ongoing education help you in applying the most current practices, but it can also be a beacon of hope for those struggling with mental health issues, as it demonstrates your commitment to their well-being and recovery.

Specializations in mental health can cater to populations such as adolescents, wherein you'll be able to understand and support the unique challenges teenagers face. Autism spectrum disorders, eating disorders, and PTSD are other areas which necessitate focused knowledge and a specialized skill set. By focusing in a specialization, you're not narrowing your horizons but honing a particular set of tools that will enable you to make significant impacts in specific areas.

How does one continue their education in this field? Advanced degree programs, such as a Master's in Psychology, Social Work, or a related counseling field, are typical routes. Moreover, many professional organizations offer specialized training courses and workshops that provide continuing education units (CEUs). These CEUs are often required to maintain your certifications and licensure, acting as both a mandate and an opportunity for growth.

However, it's not just formal education that can enhance your prowess as an MHT. Conferences, webinars, and peer-reviewed journals offer a way to engage with the most recent studies, therapeutic techniques, and case studies. Committing to reading the latest literature and engaging in scholarly discourse will keep your practice and approach modern and effective.

Remember, the first step to becoming a specialist is identifying your passion. Look back on your experiences: Is there a particular type of patient or disorder that resonates with you? The need to support and improve mental health care transcends every age, culture, and socioeconomic status, and amidst this diversity lie countless opportunities to specialize.

When considering a specialization, it's equally important to evaluate the demand for that specialty. Some areas may offer more job opportunities or higher pay, reflecting the urgent need for skilled professionals in those areas. For instance, the opioid epidemic has increased the need for mental health technicians experienced in substance abuse and addiction. Aligning your passion with societal needs not only adds meaning to your work but also ensures a relevant and rewarding career path.

Once you have completed additional training or education, it's time to showcase your new credentials. Update your resume, inform your employer, and network within your new specialty. Attend specialized meetings and join relevant professional organizations to expand your professional circle and discover new opportunities.

It's never too late or too early to commit to a lifelong learning journey. As an MHT, you're in a privileged position to affect change every day. Whether you've just entered the field or have been walking the path for years, furthering your education and specializing can reignite your passion and ensure that the care you provide is nothing short of extraordinary.

Furthering education and specialization also open doors to leadership and teaching roles. With experience and advanced knowledge, you can become a mentor to others entering the field. Teaching and passing on your expertise fits seamlessly into the ethos of mental health care, which at its heart is about helping others to grow and heal.

In a profession where burnout is a known risk, engaging in new learning opportunities can be rejuvenating. It breaks the routine and challenges you in different ways. Specializing can bring a fresh perspective to your work, make your daily routine more interesting, and help you build resilience against burnout by continuously adding new layers of expertise and interest to your career.

You might be wondering about the financial and time investments that continuing education and specializations require. It's understandable to worry about the cost, but remember, investing in your education is investing in your future. Many employers offer tuition assistance, and there are scholarships and grants specifically designed for those working in the health care sector. Always explore all your options.

In conclusion, the path of continuing education and specialization is a rich and rewarding one that can set you apart in the field of mental health care. It allows you to serve those in need with a greater depth of knowledge and to approach your work with a renewed sense of mission. It's about inspiring change, growth, and healing - not just in your patients, but within yourself, as well. Pursue your passion, expand your capabilities, and the horizons of your influence and satisfaction in your career will know no bounds.

Chapter 5:
A Day in the Life of a Mental Health Technician

Imagine the morning sun painting a warm glow across the horizon as you prepare for a day that promises both challenges and profound fulfillment. As a mental health technician, the canvas of your day is filled with a spectrum of human emotions, delicate situations, and the chance to make a real difference. From the moment you step into the facility, you tap into a well of empathy and expertise, ready to navigate the ebb and flow of patients' needs. Your daily responsibilities become a dance of routine and adaptability—monitoring patient progress, facilitating group activities, and ensuring meticulous documentation. Even your interactions are laced with purpose, as collaboration with a multidisciplinary team turns into a symphony of shared knowledge and mutual support. Every word you exchange, every act of care, upholds the highest standards of confidentiality and ethics. Each chapter of this day isn't just about the tasks at hand but about painting hope and healing into the lives of those you serve. As you lay your head down tonight, you'll know that in the heart of the mental health cosmos, your role as a technician is a beacon of unwavering dedication and transformational impact.

Daily Responsibilities and Routine

Embarking on a career as a Mental Health Technician (MHT) involves more than just possessing a desire to help others. It is a commitment to a set of daily routines and responsibilities that are both challenging and rewarding. In this richly textured landscape of mental healthcare, the tapestry of your day will be woven with the threads of routine tasks and the vibrant colors of human interaction. The daily life of an MHT is one marked by variety yet underscored by a consistent structure designed to provide the most effective support to those in need.

Each morning, as sunlight peeks through the blinds, you, the emerging MHT, will step into settings that act as both sanctuaries and spaces for healing. Your day begins by reviewing the status of patients—new notes in their charts, updates from the night staff, and any changes in medication or treatment plans. You'll be charged with understanding these nuances, for they are the guiding stars in the firmament of care you provide.

Part of the ritual will be the hand-off—a time-honored tradition in healthcare where shifts change and new faces take the helm. In these moments, keen listening is your greatest ally. You'll capture the subtle undertones of information that might be pivotal in managing the day's challenges. This isn't just about transferring information; it's about ensuring continuity and safety in a world where details matter profoundly.

As the sun climbs higher, your role as an MHT finds you performing safety checks—ensuring that the environment remains secure and that any potential hazards are swiftly addressed. Like a guardian, you oblige by the principle of 'primum non nocere'—first, do no harm. These checks, although routine, are far from mundane; they are the bulwarks that uphold the well-being of the vulnerable.

Moving through the halls, you're part observer, part doer. Your tasks include monitoring vital signs, helping with personal hygiene tasks when necessary, and aiding in mobility for those with physical limitations. These acts of service aren't merely functional; they are profound echoes of the empathy that called you to this field.

Soon, breakfast arrives, and with it, the rhythm of the day builds momentum. You assist with mealtime, which is not only a matter of nutrition but also an opportunity for social engagement and observation. You're watchful for changes in appetite or behavior—a frown, a moment of hesitation, a laugh—each is a puzzle piece in the overall emotional and mental state of your patients.

As the day unfolds, you find yourself facilitating or assisting with treatments and therapies. Whether it's setting up for group therapy, preparing materials for cognitive exercises, or offering a supportive presence during individual sessions, your role is to ensure that the therapeutic process is seamless and patient-focused.

Documentation forms the backbone of your routine. Charting progress, reporting anomalies, and logging activities—these scribbles and notes are vital cogs in the machine of mental health care. They tell a story, build a history, and inform future care. Precision and attention to detail are your allies in this task, reflective of the great responsibility entrusted to you.

Amidst these tasks, you practice active listening and observation—toolsets that are paramount. You look for non-verbal cues, shifts in mood, and moments of clarity or confusion among the patients. Each observation is an opportunity to better understand and support the healing journey, and you hold these observations in strict confidence, a sacred trust between you and those in your care.

Lunchtime is not just a break in the day; it's another chance for community and monitoring wellness. As you assist those who need help, you're also participating in an intricate dance of social dynamics, encouraging positive interaction, and maintaining a peaceful atmosphere.

In the afternoon, it's time to assist with or conduct recreational or therapeutic activities. These could range from art therapy to exercise, from journaling sessions to mindfulness practice. Here, you don't just witness transformation, you're an active participant, helping to elucidate the path forward for each individual, celebrating every step of progress.

Each moment of your day as an MHT is interspersed with opportunities to teach and encourage. Perhaps it's demonstrating proper hygiene, guiding a meditation, or simply sharing a kind word. You're not just a technician; you're an educator, a mentor, and at times, a source of inspiration.

As the day starts to wane, you prepare for the evening, helping patients wind down, ensuring they've taken their medications, and setting the stage for a restful night. A tranquil dusk in the ward is not merely a happy coincidence, but the fruit of your labor and care—the result of a day spent nurturing calm and order.

Before you pass the baton to the night shift, you'll participate in another report, this time imparting your own observations and experiences from the day. Your insights become part of the collective effort to heal and support, a testament to the collaboration that is the heart of mental health care.

Finally, as you remove your scrubs and reflect on the day, remember that each routine task carried with it the weight of someone's world. What might be a daily responsibility for you can mean a lifeline for someone else. You're not just clocking hours; you're making a tangible difference in the lives of those seeking mental wellness. Carry this knowledge with you—it's both a privilege and a potent source of motivation as you forge ahead in this noble pursuit.

Working with a Multidisciplinary Team

This lies at the heart of a mental health technician's role. As we've explored the varied aspects of this profession, let's delve into the dynamic world of collaborative health care.

Imagine you're part of an orchestra, each musician a master of their instrument. Together, you're tasked with playing a symphony, each note and rest is significant. In mental health care, a multidisciplinary team operates much like this ensemble. The psychiatrist, psychologist, nurse, social worker, and you, the mental health technician, are key players in this orchestra of wellness. Your ability to harmonize your skills with others' expertise determines the efficacy of patient care.

Working within such a team means understanding the value of each member's role. A psychiatrist may lead the treatment plan with medication management, while a psychologist provides therapeutic strategies. Nurses administer medication and monitor physical health, and social workers address external influences, such as family dynamics and community resources. Your role, as the technician on the ground, is to bring these plans to life with day-to-day patient interactions.

Communication is the linchpin of effective teamwork. Just as a slight miscommunication can disrupt a whole orchestra, a lack of clarity can cause treatment plans to falter. It's crucial that you articulate observations about patients' progress or setbacks clearly, succinctly, and professionally. In these instances, your insights provide invaluable feedback that can steer a patient's treatment plan toward success.

Respect for diversity of thought and approach within the team is also essential. Just as different instruments bring depth to music, different professional backgrounds enrich the treatment plan. Embrace the varied perspectives of your colleagues, and recognize that this diversity fosters a more holistic approach to patient care.

Conflict resolution skills come into play when disagreements arise. It's important to remain focused on the shared goal: the well-being of the patient. Approach conflicts with an open mind, a willingness to understand, and a readiness to find common ground. Sometimes, bridging differences can lead to innovative solutions.

Assertiveness paired with humility allows you to effectively advocate for patient needs while remaining open to guidance and correction. The balance between advocating for what you believe is right for a patient and being adaptable to evidence-based practices is a delicate one. You must assert yourself in advocating for patients but also understand that you are part of a larger team with a collective mission.

Understanding the scope of practice is critical in a multidisciplinary setting. You must be aware of the boundaries of your role and the expertise that others on the team bring. Crossing into areas outside your scope can lead to errors and conflict. Instead, collaborate with others to bridge gaps in care.

Developing interprofessional relationships nurtures a supportive work environment. Getting to know your colleagues not just by the services they provide but as people can open communication channels and build trust. It strengthens teamwork, ultimately improving patient outcomes.

Actively participating in team meetings is another key to successful collaboration. These forums are where treatment plans are developed, roles are defined, and patient progress is discussed. Your contributions can shed light on practical aspects of care that others may overlook.

Effective documentation is non-negotiable. It's the common thread that ensures all team members are privy to up-to-date patient information. As a technician, your thorough notes on patient behaviors, responses to treatment, and daily activities are indispensable.

Celebrating team successes bolsters team morale and personal satisfaction. Each milestone a patient reaches is a win for the entire team. Acknowledge and appreciate the collective effort, and let these triumphs fuel your passion for the work you do.

Personal development keeps you contributing effectively to the team. Pursuing additional training and staying abreast of best practices will enrich your teamwork and patient care. It benefits not only your professional growth but also the growth of your team's collective expertise.

Lastly, each member of a mental health team leans on one another for support. Recognizing the human aspect of your colleagues, that they too experience stress and emotional burden, fosters empathy within the team. Support each other, and you'll find the resilience to continue providing compassionate care.

The symphony of care you provide as a mental health technician within a multidisciplinary team is a beautiful reflection of collaboration in action. Embrace this role, for the chorus of minds and talents in harmony sets the stage for healing and the enhancement of mental health care. Each day, with each patient, you're part of a masterful ensemble making a profound difference in the lives of those you serve.

The Importance of Confidentiality and Ethics

Confidentiality and ethics in the realm of mental health care are cornerstones that should not be overlooked. As we delve into this crucial topic, let's grasp the magnitude of trust placed in the hands of Mental Health Technicians (MHTs). You, as a current or aspiring MHT, hold the keys to the private worlds of those you serve. This responsibility binds you not only legally but to a high ethical standard that upholds the dignity and respect of every individual under your care.

Confidentiality refers to the ethical principle that certain communications should be kept secret unless consent is granted for disclosure. In your role, you will be privy to sensitive information about a patient's history, condition, and treatment. It is imperative that this information remains secure, protecting patient privacy and upholding the trust essential to the therapeutic relationship. Failure to maintain confidentiality can have dire consequences, not only for the patient's well-being but also for the integrity of the mental health care system.

Ethics, on the other hand, encompasses a broader scope of professional behavior. It ensures that MHTs act with integrity, make decisions that prioritize the welfare of their patients, and commit to ongoing professional development. Ethical considerations shape the environment in which confidentiality functions, offering a framework for decision-making when faced with moral dilemmas. It's a dynamic compass that navigates the complexities of human behavior and professional responsibilities.

Understanding the legal ramifications of breaching confidentiality is non-negotiable. Laws such as the Health Insurance Portability and Accountability Act (HIPAA) in the United States provide clear guidelines on the handling of Personal Health Information (PHI). As an MHT, you must be thoroughly versed in these regulations, ensuring compliance in all aspects of patient interaction and information management.

The impact of violating confidentiality can be catastrophic—emotionally, legally, and professionally for both the patient and the technician. At the heart of the matter, such a breach can erode the therapeutic alliance necessary for effective treatment. Trust once broken can be challenging to restore, and it may compromise the mental well-being of the patient who believed their secrets were safe in a haven of healing.

Beyond legal imperatives, ethical practice entails discerning right from wrong beyond what is written in the law. Ethics empower MHTs to navigate grey areas where regulations may fall short or where individual circumstances call for nuanced judgment. It's about maintaining professional boundaries, recognizing potential conflicts of interest, and safeguarding the interests of those in vulnerable positions.

Ethical decision-making is not a static skill but an evolving process that requires reflection, consultation, and a commitment to learning. It involves understanding the values and principles that underpin mental health care and putting them into action consistently—day in and day out. MHTs often face situations that are not cut-and-dry, which is why it's essential to have a solid ethical foundation from which to operate.

The culture of confidentiality and ethics must permeate the entire mental health care team. As an MHT, you're part of a multidisciplinary force where information must often be shared for patient benefit. In such scenarios, it's vital to ensure that every team member respects the parameters of confidentiality and upholds ethical conduct.

Training in confidentiality and ethics should be ongoing. The field of mental health is ever-evolving, with new technologies like telemedicine and electronic health records presenting fresh challenges to privacy. Staying updated with current trends, best practices, and legal changes is not merely beneficial—it's essential for quality patient care and professional credibility.

Mentorship and supervision play a critical role in cultivating ethical practice. Seasoned professionals can guide you through complex situations, reinforcing ethical principles and helping you interpret them in real-life scenarios. Engaging in discussions about ethical dilemmas fosters a nuanced understanding and prepares you to act with integrity when tested.

Confidentiality breaches and ethical violations can also lead to professional sanctions, including the revocation of certifications or licenses. Your career and reputation as an MHT hinge on abiding by confidentiality and ethical codes. Protecting your professional standing is parallel to protecting your patients—each action you take, or refrain from taking, symbolizes your commitment to their welfare.

A culture of ethical practice furthers the mission of mental health care. It creates an ecosystem where patients feel secure and where practitioners can work with the assurance that their peers are equally dedicated to doing what is right. As an MHT, you're a critical component of this culture, influencing it through your actions and attitude.

The journey to becoming a trusted MHT is a testament to your character and dedication. Upholding confidentiality and ethics is not merely fulfilling a duty; it is an honor. It's a testament to your compassion and respect for the human spirit and an enduring commitment to the highest standards of care. Your role is integral in shaping a future where mental health care is synonymous with trust, dignity, and unwavering ethical conduct.

Your understanding and application of confidentiality and ethics form the bedrock of your professional identity as a Mental Health Technician. It is a sacred trust that, once embraced, elevates the standard of care for all. Let this knowledge energize and inspire you as you embark on this noble path, knowing that your adherence to these principles has the power to heal, to safeguard, and to transform lives.

Chapter 6:
Understanding the Patient Population

In harnessing the true essence of empathy and efficacy in the mental health sector, one must first cultivate a deep understanding of the varied tapestry that is the patient population. Akin to learning a new language, embracing the unique demographics and common disorders prevalent among patients is essential for fostering meaningful connections—each individual represents a singular narrative within the broader mental health narrative. Within this chapter, we delve into the layers of diversity that shape patient experiences, emphasizing the critical nature of cultural sensitivity as a cornerstone of compassionate mental health care. The art of building trust and rapport, while often overlooked, stands as a pillar in the healing journey; hence, we explore the delicate dance of establishing genuine rapport. By grasping the rich complexity of those we serve, the resolve to illuminate paths to wellness for individuals from all walks of life is not just an aim, but an imperative. Our charge is clear: to reach into the hearts of those in our care and in doing so, become vessels of transformation in their worlds as much as in our own professional odyssey.

Demographics and Common Disorders

As we transition from understanding the role of mental health technicians, it becomes imperative to grasp the demographics of those we aim to serve and the common disorders they may face. Knowledge of the varying backgrounds of patients and the prevalence of specific mental health conditions is foundational to providing empathetic and effective care. Thus, we delve into the important characterization of the patient population through demographic patterns and commonly encountered mental health challenges.

First, consider the panorama of mental health disorders, which can affect anyone irrespective of age, race, gender, or socioeconomic status. However, prevalence rates can indeed vary within these demographic segments. For instance, mood disorders such as depression have been shown to have a higher prevalence in young adults and among females than in other groups. Understanding these nuances is fundamental in anticipating and meeting the needs of distinct patient cohorts.

Anxiety disorders, including generalized anxiety disorder, social anxiety, and panic disorder, are some of the most widespread mental health issues across all demographics but tend to be more prevalent among the younger populations. Awareness of this tendency helps mental health technicians to approach their interaction with younger patients with heightened sensitivity to signs of undue stress and anxiety.

Substance use disorders often co-occur with mental health disorders and have their own demographic trends. Age and socioeconomic factors play a considerable role here, with substance abuse being more common in certain marginalized communities and among certain age groups. This reinforces the importance of a keen understanding of the socioeconomic context surrounding patients.

Among the elderly population, we notice a higher incidence of cognitive disorders such as Alzheimer's disease and other forms of dementia. Recognizing the intersection of age-related conditions with mental health is essential for mental health technicians who work with geriatric patients, as it impacts communication strategies and the nature of care provided.

Moreover, it's enlightening to examine schizophrenia's demographic footprint, which typically presents in early adulthood. Such knowledge alerts mental health technicians to be vigilant about the emergence of symptoms in patients who may be at the cusp of this age range, enabling early intervention.

Children and adolescents are not immune to mental health challenges. Disorders such as Attention-Deficit/Hyperactivity Disorder (ADHD), autism spectrum disorders, and eating disorders often first manifest in early life. With an informed background, mental health technicians can advocate for early assessments and interventions that can make a significant difference in developmental outcomes.

Gender and sexual minorities, such as those who identify as LGBTQ+, often face unique mental health challenges related to societal stigma and discrimination. This group has higher than average rates of depression, anxiety, and suicide risks. Empathetic understanding and ongoing education in cultural competency are therefore essential.

Cultural and ethnic background is another critical demographic factor influencing mental health. Socio-cultural stressors and disparities in access to healthcare contribute to the vulnerability of certain ethnic groups to mental health disorders. Mental health technicians can play an important role in bridging these gaps through culturally sensitive care and advocacy for fair access to services.

It's also pertinent to acknowledge the impact of trauma on mental health across all demographics. Disorders such as post-traumatic stress disorder (PTSD) can result from various traumatic experiences, from military combat to personal violence or abuse. Awareness and prospected care for patients with trauma histories greatly improve the possibilities of recovery and resilience.

Considering socioeconomic status, it becomes clear that individuals from lower income brackets often have higher rates of mental health disorders. This could be attributed to higher levels of stress associated with financial instability, poorer living conditions, and lack of access to quality healthcare. Mental health technicians in community settings, in particular, may encounter these complex dynamics regularly.

Geographic factors also play a role, as certain rural or underserved areas may lack mental health resources, contributing to higher rates of untreated mental illnesses. Professionals in these areas need to be resourceful, creative, and proactive in providing care and linking patients to available support structures.

In summary, mental health technicians must adopt a multifaceted lens to understand the patient population they serve. This demographic understanding, paired with knowledge of common disorders, equips you to approach each patient with the tailored care they deserve. In delivering care that recognizes the specifics of demographics and disorders, you inevitably contribute to a more equitable and effective mental health system.

As you join this vital field, remember that each statistic represents a life, each demographic slice is a collection of personal stories. Your role, your compassion, your technical skill, and your insight – these are the tools you'll wield to transform lives. You're stepping into a journey not just to witness but to actively shape the wellbeing of diverse individuals. The common threads of humanity will guide your practice, but your appreciation for the unique tapestry of each life will distinguish the care you provide.

Armed with this demographic knowledge and understanding of common disorders, you are now more prepared to encounter the rich diversity of human experiences. The challenge is not trivial, yet the rewards are profound. Taking this knowledge into your heart and hands, you will move mountains in the mental health field, one gentle, informed touch at a time.

Cultural Sensitivity in Mental Health Care

This is an essential aspect that intertwines within the fabric of mental health support. Aspiring mental health technicians must understand that every person who seeks care does so with a unique cultural background that deeply influences their perceptions, reactions, and comfort levels with the therapeutic process. It's not just about being aware of these differences—it's about actively respecting and integrating this understanding into every facet of care.

Mental health does not exist in a vacuum; it is intricately connected to cultural norms, values, and traditions. A mental health technician's ability to provide effective and empathetic care hinges on their capacity to recognize and honor these factors. This sensitivity begins with education, an open mind, and a commitment to continual learning.

Consider, for instance, the viewpoints on mental health that vary drastically across cultures. In some societies, discussing personal challenges with a stranger is taboo, while in others, mental illness may be stigmatized or misunderstood. A skilled technician can navigate these differing perspectives with grace, fostering trust and openness in the therapeutic relationship.

Cultural sensitivity also extends to communication styles. Body language, eye contact, and the way questions are phrased can all vary in meaning and acceptability. It is imperative that mental health technicians adapt their communication to respect the individual's cultural norms, allowing for clear and respectful discourse.

Fundamentally, it's about empathy—putting yourself in another's shoes. Imagine the vulnerability of sharing one's innermost thoughts and feelings. Now imagine doing this in a context where you're unsure if your cultural background will be judged or misunderstood. The security that a culturally sensitive technician offers cannot be overemphasized; it is a lifeline to those in need.

Language barriers are yet another hurdle to providing inclusive care. Translators or the use of translation services may become necessary, and technicians must be adept at working with these tools to ensure understanding and confidentiality are maintained. Misunderstandings can be detrimental, so precision in this area is crucial.

In considering treatment plans and therapeutic approaches, cultural sensitivity prompts the incorporation of diverse healing practices and beliefs. Techniques that resonate culturally can often enhance the efficacy of conventional methods, showing respect for a patient's background while promoting their well-being.

The involvement of family and community is another dimension where cultural nuances play a strong role. In some cultures, the collective well-being takes precedence over the individual, and involvement of the family in therapy may be not just preferred but expected. A mental health technician must be adept at involving these critical support systems in a way that benefits the patient's recovery.

Nutrition and lifestyle choices rooted in cultural practice also need careful consideration. Dietary restrictions or traditional remedies are integral to many people's lives, and disregarding them can alienate patients. Moreover, these aspects might even hold the key to more personalized and, therefore, more effective care strategies.

Cultural sensitivity means staying attuned to the social and political contexts that affect mental health. Discrimination, socio-economic barriers, and historical trauma all weigh heavily on a person's mental state. When technicians acknowledge these realities, they validate patients' experiences and provide them with a safe space to heal.

Training in cultural competence is not a one-time event but a career-long endeavor. It's about more than just familiarization with different cultures—it's about engaging with individuals from these cultures, seeking feedback, and being willing to adapt and improve.

Addressing one's own biases is another critical component. Everyone has biases, often unconsciously held. Mental health technicians must commit to introspection and self-awareness to minimize the impact of these biases on their work. It's a journey that requires humility and courage, as it involves confronting uncomfortable truths about oneself.

Celebrating cultural diversity within the mental health care team itself also enriches a technician's perspective. Diverse teams bring myriad viewpoints and experiences, making the care provided more holistic and well-rounded.

Finally, advocacy is a part of cultural sensitivity. A mental health technician shouldn't just be cognizant of the cultural dynamics at play—they should also advocate for systemic changes that support cultural inclusivity in all aspects of mental health care.

Cultural sensitivity in mental health care is more than just a set of protocols. It's the heart and soul of compassionate, effective treatment. It empowers patients to be fully seen and understood within their cultural context. For a mental health technician, this sensitivity isn't just professional; it's profoundly personal, reflecting a dedication to serving every individual with the dignity they deserve. It is in this fertile ground of understanding and mutual respect that healing truly begins.

Building Trust and Rapport with Patients

This forms the cornerstone of effective mental health care. As you've learned about the diverse patient populations and the cultural sensitivities involved in mental health care, it's vital to appreciate the profound impact that trust and rapport can have on therapeutic outcomes. Patients often arrive with their own histories of trauma, skepticism, or fear surrounding the healthcare system. As a mental health technician, breaking through these barriers is your first task in facilitating healing.

The foundation of trust begins with your approach to the patient. Think of it not as a checklist but as a canvas—every interaction is a brushstroke contributing to a larger picture of safety and understanding. Begin with introductions; using your name and role clearly helps to demystify your position and intentions. Extend this courtesy by asking how the patient prefers to be addressed, reinforcing their humanity and individuality right from the start.

Listening is your next powerful tool. It's not merely a matter of hearing words but understanding the feelings and meanings behind them. Remember, active listening isn't passive—it involves nodding, reaffirming, and paraphrasing to show that you are fully engaged. This demonstrates that you value their words and, by extension, their experiences and feelings.

Patient interactions should be punctuated with empathy. Empathy isn't about finding solutions immediately; it's about recognizing and validating how a person feels at this moment. Phrases like "That sounds incredibly challenging" or "I can see why you'd feel that way" create a space where a patient's emotions are acknowledged and respected.

Consistency in your behavior builds reliability. When a patient knows what to expect from you, they're more likely to feel secure in your care. This means setting and maintaining clear boundaries while being personable and accessible. Know the therapy or treatment plans and explain them with clarity, showing that you are a steady guide through their journey to wellness.

Respect privacy at all times. Privacy is a legal right, but it's also a pillar of dignity. Assure patients that their conversations and records are kept confidential. This assurance lays a strong foundation of trust, showing that you are a professional who adheres to ethical standards.

Displaying genuine curiosity about a patient's life and interests helps to personalize your interactions. This doesn't mean being intrusive; asking open-ended questions about a patient's hobbies or preferences shows them that you see them as more than their diagnosis, fostering a deeper connection.

Authenticity is key. People pick up on inauthentic behavior. Your genuineness in wanting to understand and help can set a patient at ease. This isn't to say you should be unprofessional—rather, let your human side shine within the boundaries of your professional role.

Nonverbal communication can be as loud as words. Maintaining comfortable eye contact, sitting at the patient's level, and demonstrating open body language are subtle cues that you're present and focused on them. These small gestures contribute significantly to the trust-building process.

Sharing a moment of humor, when appropriate, can be incredibly disarming and humanizing. Laughter may briefly lift the weight of a patient's struggles and can serve as a bridge to deeper mutual understanding. However, always ensure your attempts at humor are sensitive and well-timed.

Consistency in schedule can also foster trust. Being punctual and present when you say you will be demonstrates respect for their time and commitment to their care. Inconsistencies can trigger doubts and fears, while predictability can be comforting in a world that may often feel chaotic to them.

Respect a patient's autonomy. While it may be easy to see what seems best for them, it's important to involve patients in their care decisions. Respect their right to choose and support their involvement in the treatment planning. This empowerment can significantly enhance their trust in the therapeutic relationship.

Celebrate small victories with your patients. Recognizing progress, no matter how small, can be a source of motivation and a sign that you are invested in their success. This positive reinforcement can strengthen the rapport and push the healing journey forward.

Lastly, remain calm and composed, especially in times of crisis or agitation. Your stability can be a beacon during a patient's storm. Being a calm, comforting presence shows patients that they can rely on you, even in their most challenging moments, which is essential in building a relationship of trust.

To wrap up, remember that trust and rapport are dynamic; they are built and maintained over time. Your genuine, consistent, and empathetic interactions can transform a patient's experience in mental health care. By embracing these principles, you're not just performing a job—you're fundamentally enhancing someone's path to healing and showcasing the invaluable role of a mental health technician in this transformative process.

Chapter 7:
Crisis Intervention and Safety

In the pulsating heart of mental health care, the ability to respond swiftly and effectively to crises stands as a cornerstone of the Mental Health Technician's role. As we continue our exploration into this noble profession, Chapter 7 delves into the critical arena of Crisis Intervention and Safety, anchoring our understanding firmly in the real-world need for vigilance, aptitude, and skill. Here, we navigate the tumultuous waters of high-risk situations with precision, embracing de-escalation techniques that not only prevent harm but also promote an atmosphere of trust and security. The art of maintaining a safe and secure environment is not just about protocols—it's about the subtle interplay of keen observation, compassionate interaction, and decisive action geared towards safeguarding both clients and caregivers. Let's empower ourselves with the knowledge and tools necessary to transform potential chaos into managed calm, altering the course of a crisis towards a horizon of healing and stability.

Recognizing and Managing High-Risk Situations

The role of a mental health technician is as challenging as it is rewarding, often acting as the frontline in a landscape fraught with crises. High-risk situations are moments charged with the potential for harm, either to the patient, staff, or others, demanding prompt and adept management. Recognizing these situations before they escalate is a foundational skill for those in the mental health field. It involves perceptiveness, an understanding of behavioral cues, and a knowledge of the specific triggers that may lead to a crisis.

High-risk scenarios can manifest in various forms; whether it's a patient exhibiting signs of aggressive behavior, a patient experiencing severe distress over a hallucination, or someone expressing suicidal ideation, the stakes are invariably high. In any of these situations, the speed and appropriateness of a response can spell the difference between calm and chaos. Consequently, a mental health technician must be well-versed in identifying subtle shifts in mood, patterns of speech, body language, and other nonverbal cues that indicate escalating risk.

Effective communication is paramount in managing these situations. This isn't just about speaking—it's about listening actively, showing empathy, and validating a person's feelings without necessarily agreeing with their distorted perceptions. Clear, calm, and directed communication can help de-escalate a crisis, showing the patient that they are heard and understood.

In addition to recognizing and de-escalating emerging crises, a mental health technician must also know how to maintain their own safety and that of others. This includes understanding the layout of the facility, knowing the protocol for alerting security personnel or summoning assistance, and being trained in non-invasive crisis-intervention techniques. It's crucial to avoid physical confrontations unless absolutely necessary and to use the least restrictive means of maintaining safety.

Documenting events is also an essential process in managing high-risk situations. Accurate records can inform future responses, provide legal documentation, and aid in debriefing sessions that follow such events. Documentation should be detailed, objective, and completed as soon as possible after the incident to ensure accuracy and clarity.

Teamwork in these high-stakes moments cannot be overstated. No mental health technician is an island. It's the collective effort, the shared knowledge, and the support of a multidisciplinary team that often carries the day. Whether it's signaling to a colleague for support, developing individualized care plans, or debriefing post-crisis, collaboration is key.

Developing situational awareness is another facet of navigating high-risk environments successfully. This means being keenly aware of one's surroundings, the mood of the room, and the dynamics between patients. Mental health technicians must anticipate rather than just react, and this foresight is developed through experience and careful observation.

Self-awareness is also crucial. Mental health technicians must be cognizant of their own emotional reactions and biases which can influence their ability to respond effectively. Personal reflections and supervision sessions are valuable for examining these responses and learning from them.

There are times when the risk for violence is acutely high. During these moments, it is essential to maintain a calm demeanor. The mental health technician's role is to diffuse tension rather than contribute to it. This can be challenging in the face of verbal or physical threats, but a composed and professional response is necessary to prevent the escalation of violence.

Knowing when to implement restrictive interventions is a significant aspect of managing crises. This should always be a last resort, used only when all other de-escalation strategies have failed and a real risk of harm exists. The use of restraints or seclusion must always comply with legal standards and ethical guidelines.

Post-crisis reflection is another critical component. Understanding what happened, why it happened, and how the response could be improved is paramount in learning from these situations. Reflecting as a team can yield insights that can refine the protocols and approaches for managing future crises.

Training and continuous education play a significant role in preparing mental health technicians to handle such high-risk scenarios confidently. Regular workshops, simulations, and role-play exercises can help reinforce crisis intervention skills and keep staff updated on best practices.

Understanding personal limits is also essential. At times, a mental health technician might identify signs that they are becoming overwhelmed. Recognizing and addressing these signs, and seeking assistance when necessary, can prevent personal distress from interfering with the care provided to patients.

Mental health technicians must also be prepared for the aftermath of a high-risk situation. Despite the best efforts, outcomes can sometimes be less than favorable. It's vital to have access to support systems and stress-relief outlets, such as debriefing with peers, speaking to a counselor, or engaging in activities outside of work that promote mental well-being.

Ultimately, managing high-risk situations is a balance of art and science. It's a symphony of employing proven strategies while customizing the approach to individual circumstances. This deep and meaningful work demands a blend of critical thinking, emotional fortitude, and a passionate commitment to service. Aspiring mental health technicians must embrace their role in shaping this intricate tapestry, where each thread represents a life touched, a crisis averted, and a community strengthened.

De-escalation Techniques and Preventing Harm

In the realm of mental health care, mental health technicians are often on the front lines, interacting with individuals in varying states of distress. The ability to de-escalate a potentially volatile situation is essential. This ability not only ensures the safety of the patient but that of the technician and others within the environment as well. De-escalation isn't just a set of actions; it's an art that combines communication, understanding, intuition, and intervention. It underscores the technician's role in fostering a stable and therapeutic setting—where healing, rather than harm, is paramount.

The first step in effective de-escalation is recognizing the signs of escalation. Tense body language, increased agitation, raised voice—these indicators can signal a need for intervention. Mental health technicians must be astute observers, attuned to the subtleties of their patients' behaviors, and proactive in addressing tensions before they escalate into physical confrontations.

Once potential for escalation has been identified, the art of communication takes center stage. Your voice, a powerful tool, should emanate calm, consistency, and compassion. By modulating tone and volume, you can create an atmosphere of understanding. Convey empathy by validating the individual's feelings without necessarily agreeing with their behavior. This validation can be profoundly calming and can reinforce the person's sense of self-worth and dignity.

Listening skills are just as vital—they let you understand the underlying issues driving the escalation. Engage in active listening, which encompasses not only hearing the words but also the emotions behind them. This will allow you to respond appropriately, addressing not just the surface-level concerns but the deep-seated needs that may be contributing to the current situation.

A key technique in de-escalation is setting boundaries with clarity and respect. Illustrating these limits helps patients understand the framework within which they can safely operate. It also establishes a sense of order and predictability, which can be particularly comforting for those feeling out of control. Make sure boundaries are consistent with overall treatment goals and communicated clearly to prevent misunderstandings.

In conjunction with verbal techniques, nonverbal cues play a significant role. Your body language should project openness and non-threatening intent. Maintain appropriate eye contact—not too intense, as this can be seen as confrontational, but enough to demonstrate your engagement and presence. The physical space between you and the patient is also crucial; provide enough distance to avoid crowding, which can be an additional stressor.

When it comes to preventing harm, proactive measures are your best defense. This includes creating an environment that minimizes triggers. Familiarize yourself with each patient's history and possible stressors, and work to mitigate these in their surroundings. Removing unnecessary stimuli that could provoke an escalation is a preventive step often overlooked, yet it can be remarkably effective.

Remember that the ability to remain calm in the face of someone else's storm is not just a skill—it is a superpower. It demonstrates to patients that no matter how chaotic their internal or external world becomes, there is a mooring point—the steadiness that you, as their technician, can offer. Arnold Toynbee once said, "The supreme accomplishment is to blur the lines between work and play." Infuse elements of ease and lightness into your interactions when appropriate to alleviate tension and model coping through calmness.

Your response to conflict should always be measured, tapping into techniques steeped in evidence-based practices. Crisis intervention training often covers various de-escalation tactics and can be invaluable in preparing you for the unexpected. Continuous learning and role-playing scenarios can bolster your confidence and competence in de-escalation skills.

Predict and manage your own emotional responses as well. It can't be understated how much your composure can influence the outcome of a stressful situation. Respond, don't react—take the space you need to gather your thoughts and emotions before you engage. Self-awareness is key; recognizing your triggers and stress responses allows you to manage them and remain focused on the individual in need.

It's imperative to know when to call for support. De-escalation is a team effort—your colleagues can offer additional strategies or simply serve as a stabilizing presence. In times of crisis, the collective effort of a well-coordinated team can make a substantial difference in the outcome. Prioritize communication with your team to ensure everyone is on the same page and can respond in unison.

Documenting any incidents thoroughly is crucial for several reasons. It helps to create an accurate record, aides in formulating future prevention strategies, and is essential for legal and ethical considerations. It also serves as a learning tool for you and your team, allowing for reflection and refinement of techniques.

Finally, debriefing after a crisis is an often underutilized, yet essential, component of prevention. Review what occurred, what was effective, and how the team can improve for future interactions. Acknowledge the emotional impact that these events can have on you and your colleagues, and ensure that support is available for those who need it.

In the journey of becoming a mental health technician, acquiring de-escalation skills is a profound testament to your dedication to serving those in need. It's a pledge to foster safety, to make room for healing, and to embody the compassionate presence that can be the difference between harm and recovery. Remember, in their search for light, your calm might just be the beacon that guides them through the darkness.

Immersing yourself in the study and practice of these techniques positions you as a pillar in the mental health community. With dedication, patience, and the courage to face adversity with a steady hand, you will not only prevent harm but also promote healing, growth, and a renewed sense of hope in the lives of those you serve.

Maintaining a Safe and Secure Environment

Safety and security form the foundation upon which all effective mental health care is built. As mental health technicians, you hold a key responsibility to uphold and maintain a secure environment that supports the well-being and recovery of those in your care. This is not merely about locks on doors and routine checks; it involves an understanding of human behavior, an awareness of one's surroundings, and the implementation of best practices to mitigate risks daily.

Your role will often require you to be the first line of defense against potential hazards. It can vary from environmental safety measures to the identification of personal risks among the patient population. To excel, you'll need to be vigilant, proactive, and knowledgeable about the facility's specific protocols and be able to adapt quickly to evolving situations.

One aspect of environmental safety is in the careful layout and furnishing of patient areas. Consider the physical space where patients spend their time. Is the furniture safe and secured? Are potentially harmful objects out of reach? The physical setting must not only be comfortable but also minimize the opportunities for a patient to harm themselves or others.

Creating a secure environment also involves regular risk assessments of the facility itself. Inspect for and address any structural dangers or malfunctioning equipment that could pose risks. Ensure that emergency exits are well marked and clear of obstructions. Regular drills and the practice of evacuation procedures are crucial to prepare staff and patients for any unexpected emergencies.

Monitoring and controlling access to the facility is another crucial component. Whether it's managing visitor access or ensuring that staff are properly credentialed, strict entry protocols can prevent unauthorized or potentially dangerous individuals from entering sensitive areas.

Personal safety of both patients and staff is paramount. Training in nonviolent de-escalation techniques is essential to handle incidents calmly and assertively. Moreover, techniques such as therapeutic communication can often prevent tension from escalating to a physical level, thus securing a peaceful resolution most of the time.

An area that requires special attention is medication management. Medications must be stored securely and administered accurately. Mismanagement of medication not only has legal ramifications but can also result in severe harm to patients. Therefore, mental health technicians must be meticulous and systematic in their approach to this aspect of care.

Documentation plays a significant role in maintaining safety and security. Incident reports, patient records, and logs of daily checks should be kept up-to-date. Accurate record-keeping allows for the tracking of patterns that may indicate rising risks and helps ensure appropriate responses are documented and learned from.

Cameras and alarm systems can provide an extra layer of security in patient care areas. However, one must balance safety with respect for privacy. Staff should be trained on the appropriate use of surveillance equipment and the legal implications of privacy violations.

Continuous education is vital to remain current with safety protocols and procedures. New threats can emerge, and regulations can change, so it's crucial for you to stay informed through webinars, workshops, and ongoing training sessions.

Collaboration with law enforcement and first responders is necessary for managing extreme cases that exceed the capabilities of the facility. Having a protocol for when and how to involve external authorities ensures that situations can be managed swiftly with the least disruption.

Finally, psychological safety should not be overlooked. Mental health facilities should be havens where stigmatization, bullying, and harassment are not tolerated. Fostering a culture of respect and safety is as essential to recovery as the medical treatment provided.

Remember, safety is everyone's responsibility. It thrives in a climate of collaboration where each team member feels empowered to speak up about potential concerns. A successful mental health technician must believe in this value and work together with colleagues to weave a tight safety net for all within the mental health care setting.

By adhering to these principles and striving to nurture a safe and secure environment, you are not only protecting the individuals in your care but are also supporting their therapeutic journey. This, in turn, contributes to a more effective and fulfilling practice. You are, after all, creating a space not just where people are housed, but where healing can truly begin.

Your conviction, paired with the knowledge and application of safety measures, stands as the bulwark against the unpredictable tidal waves of challenges that the mental health field can bring. As you make your indelible mark on this vital sector, remember that the safety and security you uphold today pave the way for the trust and healing that build the pillars of robust mental health support for tomorrow.

Chapter 8:
The Therapeutic Environment

As we journey further into the heart of mental health care, Chapter 8 invites us to explore the foundations of 'The Therapeutic Environment'—a term that transcends mere physical space to comprise a symbiotic blend of atmosphere, ethos, and action. A well-constructed therapeutic environment is an unrivaled protagonist in the narrative of healing. It harmonizes the sensory experiences with the psychological needs of the patient, cultivating a milieu where recovery can not only take root but flourish. An adept Mental Health Technician recognises that every element, from lighting and layout to the wavelengths of color adorning the walls, resonates with the psyche of those seeking solace and strength within them. Utilizing an array of therapeutic modalities, they articulate the unsung language of healing spaces. And let's not forget the pivotal role that structured recreation and activity programs play, transforming mundane moments into gateways of growth. They are the architects of ambiance, sculpting environments that uplift, empower, and ultimately, manifest as the cornerstone of therapeutic triumph.

Creating a Healing Space

Within the realm of mental health care, the environment in which healing transpires is just as paramount as the treatment itself. For a Mental Health Technician, understanding how to create a therapeutic and healing space is a core component of the facilitation of wellness. It encompasses not merely the physical environment but also the intangible atmosphere that soothes the mind and eases the soul of individuals who are facing emotional tribulations.

The first step in curating such a space is considering the physical components—a blend of comfort, safety, and aesthetic appeal. It's essential to recognize the importance of a clean, well-maintained area that feels welcoming and secure. Why? Because the environment can have a profound impact on a person's state of mind. Integrating elements like soft lighting, comfortable seating, and calming colors can significantly lower anxiety and stress levels, preparing the stage for effective therapy.

But the creation of a healing space extends beyond what the eye sees. It's about fostering a sense of trust and serenity. As a mental health technician, your demeanor can heavily influence the atmosphere. Displaying a calm and patient attitude will resonate through the room, offering reassurance to those present. Often, the emotional climate set by staff is the cornerstone from which recovery begins.

Privacy and confidentiality are the bedrocks of trust in any therapeutic setting. When creating a healing space, it's vital to ensure that conversations cannot be overheard and that patients feel their disclosures are respected and protected. This is not just about following laws and regulations—it's about honoring the inherent dignity of every individual who seeks help.

Accessibility is another crucial aspect of creating a healing space. It must be inclusive, taking into account people with different physical abilities and ensuring that accommodations are available. This consideration speaks volumes to the respect and equality afforded to all patients, regardless of their challenges.

In creating a healing environment, the subtle nuances matter. This can mean having tissues available, maintaining an organized space clear of clutter, and ensuring that any resources or materials are easily accessible. These details, though small, contribute to a patient's sense of order and peace.

A healing space is also dynamic, adapting to the varied needs and preferences of its users. Flexibility in the arrangement of furniture and the ability to personalize the space, when appropriate, can empower patients and make them feel more at ease. This adaptability should extend to sensory elements like temperature control and the option for background music or silence, according to individual treatment plans.

The influence of nature should not be underestimated in the design of a therapeutic environment. The inclusion of plants, access to natural light, or even artworks depicting serene landscapes can enhance connectedness to the outside world and provide a calming effect on patients navigating mental health challenges. It's this connection to life and growth that subliminally reinforces the journey of healing.

While aesthetics are vital, so is functionality. Every element of the space should have a purpose that aligns with therapeutic goals. From ensuring confidentiality with soundproof walls to strategically placing furniture to encourage openness and discourse, the functionality of each aspect needs to support the overarching mission of mental wellness.

Handling technology and equipment with care is equally important in creating a healing space. The sounds and sights of medical equipment can be intimidating, so integrating such devices in a way that is unobtrusive and 'humanized' can lessen any potential for further stress.

On the subject of humanization, personal touches like artwork created by patients, a community board featuring positive messages, and photographs that evoke warmth and humanity can transform a clinical space into one that is representative of collective hopes and aspirations.

Creating a healing space is also about building a community. Encourage interaction amongst patients where suitable, with communal areas designed to foster a sense of belonging and togetherness. Group activities that promote camaraderie and shared experiences can be integral to recovering individuals seeking connections with others who understand their struggles.

Yet, remember that solitude can also be healing. Sometimes, patients will require areas where they can be alone with their thoughts, to reflect or meditate. A versatile healing space will cater to this need with quiet corners or private nooks that still feel secure under the watchful and caring presence of mental health staff.

Finally, remember that a healing space is always evolving. Seek feedback from patients and colleagues, and be open to making changes that can further enhance the therapeutic environment. Continual improvement is a sign of dedication to the critical mission of healing and the drive towards excellence in mental health care.

The creation of a healing space is an ongoing, mindful process that requires attention to both the seen and unseen needs of those in mental health care. As a Mental Health Technician, your role in developing such an environment is fundamental. Every day, you have the power to impact lives profoundly, transforming spaces into sanctuaries of recovery and hope.

Implementing Therapeutic Modalities

Within the domain of mental healthcare, the integration of therapeutic modalities forms the bedrock of what mental health technicians do daily. Implementing these modalities encompasses a blend of scientific knowledge and compassionate application, requiring technicians to be both technically proficient and emotionally intelligent. At the heart of this intricate dance lies the goal of restoring, maintaining, and enhancing the mental health of individuals.

Therapeutic modalities are varied, each offering a unique approach to addressing mental health concerns. Cognitive-behavioral therapy (CBT), dialectical behavior therapy (DBT), psychodynamic therapy, and supportive counseling are just a few examples of the types of therapies that mental health technicians may facilitate or assist with. Understanding when and how to implement these modalities involves an application of both the art and science of mental health.

First, let's consider the lay of the land. Each patient presents with unique needs, so a tailored approach is critical. Mental health technicians must work closely with mental health professionals to ensure that the chosen modality aligns with the patient's diagnosis, treatment plan, and personal preferences. Collaboration within the treatment team is vital to ensuring that the implementation of any therapeutic modality is both appropriate and consistent.

Documentation is a crucial element of implementing therapeutic modalities. As a technician, you'll be tasked with meticulously recording patient responses to various interventions. These documents become a part of the patient's medical record and serve as a vital tool for tracking progress, adjusting strategies, and communicating with other members of the healthcare team. Attention to detail and a commitment to accuracy are non-negotiable traits for this aspect of the role.

Technological literacy is increasingly important in the modern mental health field, as digital platforms are often used to deliver therapies. Whether it's teletherapy sessions or computer-assisted cognitive training exercises, mental health technicians need to be competent in managing and troubleshooting these technologies, ensuring that the therapeutic process is as smooth as possible for both the practitioner and the patient.

A significant aspect of implementing therapeutic modalities is the creation of a therapeutic alliance. This term describes the partnership and level of trust between the practitioner and the patient. Mental health technicians facilitate this by setting a tone of empathy, non-judgment, and professionalism within each interaction. Your ability to listen actively, validate feelings, and offer support is invested in every moment you spend with patients.

In the pursuit of effective therapeutic outcomes, mental health technicians must also recognize the role of evidence-based practice. This means staying informed about the latest research and proven interventions, and possibly pursuing ongoing education or professional development opportunities to stay current. This commitment to learning not only enhances your qualifications but also provides patients with the most effective care.

Therapeutic boundaries must be carefully navigated. Despite the close and caring relationships that may develop, maintaining professionalism is essential. A mental health technician who understands and respects the necessary separation between themselves and their patients can foster a healthy therapeutic relationship without risking ethical violations or emotional entanglement.

Multiple therapeutic modalities can be incorporated into holistic care approaches. For instance, a patient receiving CBT for anxiety might also benefit from mindfulness exercises or physical activity programs to manage physiological symptoms. What's crucial is that each modality complements the other, and that the technician assists in coordinating these efforts.

Adaptation is key; what works for one patient might not work for another, and sometimes what worked last week isn't effective this week. Mental health technicians must stay observant, flexible, and responsive to shifting needs, ready to adjust their approach in consultation with the treatment team. It's this flexibility that allows for personalized and responsive care, a hallmark of quality mental health treatment.

Risk assessment is part of the implementation process, ensuring that any new therapeutic modality doesn't put the patient at risk of harm. Integrated into this is the management of any adverse reactions or crises that may arise during therapy. Mental health technicians are often the frontline observers of such incidents and therefore need to be trained in identifying and responding to potential risks promptly.

Cultural sensitivity is intrinsic to successfully implementing therapeutic modalities. Given the diverse backgrounds of patients, technicians must be adept at modifying delivery methods to respect cultural norms, languages, and beliefs. This cultural proficiency not only enhances mutual respect but also ensures that care is both effective and meaningful to each individual.

Aiding in the implementation of therapeutic modalities does involve managing logistics – be it scheduling sessions, preparing therapy rooms, or ensuring that resources are readily available. These administrative tasks, though sometimes mundane, are essential components that support the therapeutic process.

Lastly, self-awareness and reflection are valuable tools for a mental health technician. Reflecting on the outcomes of therapy sessions, your role in them, and the effectiveness of different modalities contributes to both personal growth and professional development. This self-assessment aligns perfectly with a career where success is measured by the profound effect on the lives of others.

Your journey as a mental health technician is one of profound meaning and impact. By understanding and implementing therapeutic modalities, you join a workforce dedicated to positive change, to the healing of minds, and to the betterment of lives. Take this task to heart, for through your hands, the world of mental health care evolves and advances toward a future of hope and healing.

The Role of Recreation and Activity in Mental Health

This a topic that burgeons with potential and necessitates a deep dive into its practical applications within the sphere of mental health care. When we look at the landscape of therapeutic modalities, it's clear that the incorporation of recreation and activities isn't a mere add-on, but a powerful cornerstone in the architecture of holistic mental health support and rehabilitation.

Recreation and structured activities are essential in engendering a sense of normalcy and joy in patients' lives. Mental health technicians will find that suggesting and facilitating such activities are an effective way to promote engagement, improve mood, and give patients a sense of control over their environment. Moreover, for individuals struggling with mental health issues, the predictability and routine that activities provide can be a soothing contrast to the chaos they may experience internally.

Fostering social interactions through group activities is also paramount. It acts not only as a way to combat the isolation often felt in mental health struggles but also helps in building a supportive community amongst patients. As social beings, our mental health is intricately linked with the relationships we maintain and cultivate. By skillfully navigating group dynamics, technicians can instill a sense of belonging – a vital ingredient for mental well-being.

Moreover, when we talk about mental health, we often focus on the mind, sometimes overlooking the profound interconnectedness of the mind and body. Physical activities, be it sports, dance, or yoga, can be tremendously beneficial. They are more than just exercise; they serve as non-verbal outlets for emotional expression and stress relief. They release endorphins, often termed as 'nature's mood lifters', fostering an improved mental state.

Another critical aspect is the concept of mastery and accomplishment that comes with learning new skills or engaging in activities. When patients learn to play a musical instrument, paint, or cook in a therapeutic setting, they not only enrich their skillset but also their confidence and self-esteem. It's a victory they can own, and that sense of achievement can ignite hope and the courage to tackle other challenges in their recovery journey.

Engagement in creative endeavors like art, drama, or writing workshops offers a safe space for expression and processing complex emotions. It's where words may fail, but colors, shapes, and narratives succeed in telling the story of a patient's inner world. The role of a mental health technician in facilitating such therapeutic activities is to guide patients in exploring these mediums as a language for their emotions – empowering them to communicate and understand themselves better.

Activities also provide structure to a patient's day. This can be critical for those whose mental health symptoms can result in disorganization or a feeling of being overwhelmed by unstructured time. Structured activity programs give patients the opportunity to practice tasks and schedules that are similar to those they would encounter in everyday life, thereby enhancing their ability to function outside the therapeutic environment.

Additionally, engagements in activities can be tailored to individual interests, further personalizing the care approach and promoting adherence to treatment plans. Personalization ensures that the activities not only fit the unique needs but also tap into the inherent strengths and passions of the patients, making the therapeutic process more enjoyable and effective.

In the process of engaging patients in these activities, a mental health technician also has the opportunity to observe. Observation can give key insights into a patient's progress, areas of difficulty, social interactions, and much more. These observations can inform the broader treatment strategy and adjustments that may be required.

Harnessing the power of nature through ecotherapy or horticultural activities can be profoundly healing as well. Working with plants or being outdoors can reduce feelings of anger, stress, and depression. It's less about the act of gardening and more about reconnecting with the cycle of life and a sense of purpose and caretaking.

Recreation and activity are not stand-alone treatments but should be considered an integral part of a multi-modal intervention strategy. When combined with other therapeutic approaches like medication, psychotherapy, or cognitive behavioral therapy, they offer a synergistic effect, each component amplifying the healing impact of the other.

It's important to note, however, that while recreation and activities offer numerous benefits, mental health technicians must also be mindful of the potential for overstimulation or exacerbation of symptoms in certain individuals. Knowing when to facilitate or when to scale back is a nuanced skill that technicians must develop through experience and observation.

Mental health technicians play a crucial role in advocating for and enabling access to recreational activities. They act as liaisons between the patients and the therapeutic offerings, and they must possess the discernment to match activities to the therapeutic goals and the individual's needs. The technician's enthusiasm and genuine belief in the transformative potential of these activities can be infectious, creating a more receptive and motivated patient.

This role comes with the responsibility of being culturally sensitive and aware of various forms of recreation that may resonate with distinct cultural backgrounds. It's about creating a space that feels inclusive and representative of the diversity of interests and cultural expressions of the patient population.

As we continue to explore and understand the vast terrains of mental health, the importance of putting theories into action is paramount. Remember, it's in the application - in the hands-on experience where we truly learn, adapt, and see the fruits of our labor. Incorporating recreation and activities in mental health care is more than a job; it's a pursuit of passion, creativity, and a deep commitment to facilitating the joy and enrichment in the lives of those we serve.

Chapter 9:
Legal and Ethical Considerations

Embarking on a journey into mental health as a technician carries with it not just the opportunity to make a profound impact on the lives of those you'll serve, but also the responsibility to navigate the complex web of legal and ethical frameworks designed to protect both patients and practitioners. This chapter serves as your compass through the terrain where patient rights intersect with the duty of care, where confidentiality transcends into a sanctuary of trust, and where professional boundaries are not barriers but the very foundations upon which therapeutic relationships thrive. As you stride forward, remember that the conduct you exhibit and the decisions you make echo the core values of this noble profession. Here, you'll learn to distill clarity from ethical dilemmas—not solely arming yourself with the rules from textbooks but honing the moral intuition that will guide you through the gray. Embrace this knowledge; let it fortify your resolve, for it's not just about adhering to laws—it's about embodying the virtues that define the heart of mental health care.

Patient Rights and Confidentiality

Understanding the sanctity of patient rights and confidentiality is a cornerstone of mental health care. As a prospective or budding mental health technician, fully grasping these principles is essential not only for legal adherence but also for building trust with your patients. Reflect on this: The relationships you foster with those under your care may well be the highlight of their day, or even a lifeline in moments of profound turmoil. Let this magnitude inspire you as we explore the delicate fabric of patient rights and confidentiality.

Your journey in mental health care will introduce you to people from all walks of life, each with their own stories, struggles, and triumphs. As a mental health technician, you're entrusted with sensitive information that, if disclosed improperly, could have severe repercussions for the individuals in your care. It's imperative to understand that confidentiality isn't just a best practice—it's a patient's right, protected under laws like the Health Insurance Portability and Accountability Act (HIPAA) in the United States.

Confidentiality extends beyond protecting health records; it encompasses respecting the privacy of individuals' thoughts, feelings, and experiences shared within the therapeutic environment. Imagine yourself as a guardian of secrets, a role that demands integrity and discretion at all times. Remember, when a patient confides in you, they're not just sharing information—they're handing you a piece of their vulnerability, relying on your professionalism to safeguard it.

However, understanding patient confidentiality also involves recognizing exceptions to the rule. There will be moments when you must balance confidentiality with safety, such as when a patient is at risk of harming themselves or others. This ethical tightrope requires you to be both knowledgeable about mandatory reporting laws and compassionate in your approach. It's about doing what's right for the patient while adhering to the legal framework that guides your profession.

The concept of "minimum necessary" should become second nature to you. This principle means that you only access and disclose the least amount of personal information required to perform your job effectively. It's a subtle, yet significant way of honoring a patient's privacy and reinforcing the protective boundaries around their personal health information.

Moreover, patient rights extend to their autonomy and involvement in their care. As a technician, you'll facilitate patients' rights to make informed decisions about their treatment options. This requires clear communication, fostering understanding, and actively supporting a person's right to consent or refuse treatment. It's about empowering patients, ensuring their voices are heard, and their choices respected.

Part of respecting patient rights is adhering to the principles of informed consent. This means going beyond obtaining a signature on a form—it's an ongoing process of ensuring that patients understand the purpose, benefits, risks, and alternatives to the treatments or interventions they're offered. Informed consent is an active dialogue, an invitation to engage patients as participants in their health journey, not mere bystanders.

In your role, you'll navigate the subtleties of capacity and consent. Some individuals may have cognitive limitations or conditions that impact their ability to make decisions. Here, your sensitivity and ability to assess decision-making capacity become vital, often involving collaboration with family members, guardians, or legal representatives while still prioritizing the patient's preferences and dignity.

Recording and handling patient information are tasks that demand meticulous attention to detail. Whether electronic or paper-based, the systems you use will require vigilance to prevent unauthorized access. Your actions, from logging out of computers to locking file cabinets, contribute to a culture of confidentiality that protects both your patients and your workplace.

Training and education are your allies in maintaining confidentiality. Your employer will likely provide specific guidelines and protocols, but it's your responsibility to remain current with evolving regulations and practices. Continuous learning, asking questions when in doubt, and participating in training sessions will ensure you uphold the highest standards of privacy.

Rapport and trust-building are at the heart of mental health care. A patient's knowledge that their rights are recognized and their information is protected enhances their sense of safety and can significantly improve therapeutic outcomes. Be the technician who patients feel they can trust, one who recognizes the human behind the health record and treats their rights with the utmost respect.

Conversations around confidentiality should also permeate your interactions with colleagues. While teamwork and collaboration are critical, discussing patient information should be confined to professional contexts where it's necessary for care coordination. Casual conversations or curiosity have no place in the discussion of a patient's personal health matters.

An ethical conundrum may arise when the interests of the patient seem to conflict with broader societal concerns. In such situations, you must navigate the complexities with wisdom and seek guidance from supervisors or ethics committees. Your ethical compass must be finely attuned to the nuances of each unique scenario, ensuring you act in a manner that's both legally sound and morally upright.

Upholding patient rights and confidentiality isn't just about following rules; it's about fostering a healing atmosphere where patients feel valued and protected. Carry with you the understanding that each act of protection is an affirmation of your patients' humanity and that each gesture of respect contributes to their wellness journey.

As a future mental health technician, let the gravity and beauty of this responsibility ignite your passion for service. Remember, patient rights and confidentiality are more than just legal obligations; they are the pillars upon which the sacred space of healing is built. Hold these tenets close as you embark on this noble path, championing the dignity and respect every individual deserves.

Professional Boundaries and Conduct

In the landscape of mental health care, mental health technicians serve as a cornerstone, providing essential support to individuals facing mental health challenges. The nature of this support is intricate, blurring lines between personal empathy and professional detachment. Navigating these waters requires a sound understanding of professional boundaries and conduct, which ensures the safety and well-being of both the patient and the technician.

Establishing clear professional boundaries is crucial. These not only protect the patient's confidentiality and right to privacy but also secure the mental health technician's position as a trustworthy and ethical caregiver. Boundaries are the defined limits that separate the therapeutic behavior of a professional from any other behavior that could reduce the benefit of care to patients.

It's essential to recognize that while warmth and empathy are powerful healing tools in mental health care, they should not compromise the professional relationship. Personal relationships with patients, for example, can lead to conflicts of interest, bias in treatment decisions, and can even result in harm to the patient or the professional's career.

Social media and digital communication have added a layer of complexity to professional boundaries. Technicians must be particularly cautious, maintaining professionalism online just as they would in person. This means being mindful of privacy settings, not engaging in personal conversations with patients, and understanding that the digital footprint you leave could impact your professional reputation.

Professional conduct extends beyond boundaries with patients to include interactions with colleagues and the multidisciplinary team. Mental health technicians must foster an environment of mutual respect and clear communication. Harassment, discrimination, or any form of unprofessional behavior can not only destabilize the team dynamic but also detract from patient care.

Dual relationships, or multiple roles, pose significant risks in mental health settings. These occur when a technician has another role with a patient, whether it be as a friend, family member, business associate, or romantic partner. These relationships can obscure clarity, introduce bias, and potentially lead to clinical decisions that are not in the best interest of the patient.

The maintenance of confidentiality is another critical component of professional conduct. Sharing patient information without consent (unless mandated by law) is not just unethical; it is illegal. Mental health technicians must be conversant with the laws and regulations governing patient privacy and confidentiality, including the Health Insurance Portability and Accountability Act (HIPAA).

In situations where the line between personal and professional becomes cloudy, supervision and consultation play essential roles. Seeking advice from more experienced colleagues or supervisors when faced with ethical uncertainties can provide clarity and reinforce the importance of maintaining professional boundaries.

Documentation is another key aspect of professional conduct. Accurate, timely, and thorough documentation of patient interactions not only aids in ensuring quality care but also serves as a legal record. It is a testament to the technician's professionalism and attention to detail.

Maintaining an ongoing commitment to professional development and education is fundamental to professional conduct. As laws, technologies, and best practices evolve, so must the knowledge base of the mental health technician. This commitment to learning reflects a dedication to quality care and an acknowledgement of the evolving nature of mental health care.

Gifts and tokens of gratitude from patients can present complex situations. It's important to handle such instances with sensitivity while adhering to the facility's policies to ensure there is no misinterpretation of motives or compromise to the professional relationship.

When faced with challenging patients or situations that test your patience and resilience, it's imperative to remember that professional conduct includes composure and the ability to manage one's emotions. Responding with kindness, yet firmly, helps maintain order and safety in what can often be a volatile setting.

Lastly, self-awareness is a crucial component of professional conduct. Understanding your own boundaries, emotional triggers, and personal biases allows you to navigate the caregiver role more effectively. It underpins the ability to provide consistent, compassionate care while sustaining personal integrity and job satisfaction.

As you move forward on this path, let these principles of professional boundaries and conduct guide your steps. They are not just rules to follow, but pillars that uphold the noble cause you serve. Recognize your role as both a beacon of professionalism and a guardian of your patients' journey toward mental well-being. Embrace it with the gravitas and grace it demands, for in doing so, you become not just a technician, but a vital part of the healing process.

In conclusion, remember that every interaction in the realm of mental health care is an opportunity to reinforce trust, demonstrate competence, and uphold the dignity of the profession. As a mental health technician, you are an embodiment of the standards you practice, making it crucial to adopt a conscientious approach towards boundaries and conduct that resonates with the core values of care, respect, and ethics.

Navigating Ethical Dilemmas

As a mental health technician, you are bound to face a myriad of ethical dilemmas that test your integrity, judgment, and the application of your knowledge. The path through these dilemmas is rarely clear-cut, and it is a terrain where one must tread with both a strong moral compass and a flexible, open mind. Let's explore the strategies for successfully navigating the sometimes rock-strewn road of ethical quandaries.

Your role as a mental health technician will often require you to act as a gatekeeper, responsible for the welfare of those under your care. During these times, you'll find that textbook solutions don't always fit real-life situations. How can you discern the right course of action? It's essential to start with the foundational values of mental health care: respect for the autonomy of the patient, the promotion of their best interests, nonmaleficence, and justice.

Understanding ethical principles is a singular piece of the puzzle. It's in the synthesis of these principles with professional guidelines where effective resolution of ethical dilemmas begins. Professional codes of conduct, which provide a framework for addressing issues that arise, should be well known to you. Familiarize yourself with the American Counseling Association's Code of Ethics, the National Association of Psychiatric Health Systems' guidelines, or other relevant standards that align with your role.

When you come face to face with an ethical dilemma, it's beneficial to have a systematic approach to problem-solving. Identify the problem clearly, consider the context, consult the relevant ethical standards, and reflect on the potential outcomes of your decisions. Remember, in some cases, your decisions can have far-reaching implications, affecting not only the patient's life but also the wider community.

Teamwork and collaboration can be invaluable when unraveling an ethical knot. Seeking the counsel of colleagues, supervisors, or an ethics committee within your organization can provide new perspectives and seasoned insight. These discussions encourage an environment where different viewpoints are appreciated and can lead you to a more considered and appropriate solution.

One of the most challenging aspects of ethical dilemmas is when they involve a conflict between a patient's wishes and their well-being. For instance, a patient might refuse medication that is critical to their recovery. Here, your ability to engage in effective communication is crucial. Can you find a way to respect their autonomy while also acting in their best interest? Sometimes, finding a compromise or presenting alternate solutions may resolve such an ethical standoff.

Confidentiality is another cornerstone of mental health care that often presents ethical challenges. Maintaining a patient's privacy is paramount, but what if you learn of a situation where keeping this confidentiality could lead to harm? Balancing the duty to protect a patient's information with the responsibility to prevent harm to the individual or others is a moral tightrope that requires care and expertise.

Documentation is also a critical component of ethical practice. Keeping precise, accurate records not only supports clinical care but also provides a clear account of decisions and interventions, which is vital should there be a need to review an ethical decision. Always document your ethical decision-making process, including the consultations and considerations that informed your actions.

Sensitivity to cultural differences is essential when addressing ethical dilemmas. What might be an acceptable practice in one culture could be taboo in another. A culturally informed approach to care involves recognizing these differences and adapting your approach accordingly, without compromising ethical standards.

In the event of a mistake or oversight on your part, it is paramount to confront the issue directly. Ethical practice demands accountability. Transparent communication with your supervisors and colleagues, acknowledging the error, and taking steps to rectify it is crucial to maintaining trust and credibility within your team and with your patients.

Self-care comes into play in navigating ethical dilemmas as well. The stress of resolving these issues can wear on you, so it's important to be cognizant of the impact and engage in practices that maintain your well-being. Allowing yourself to debrief with colleagues or a supervisor after a particularly difficult case can be tremendously helpful in processing the situation.

While the field continuously evolves and you encounter new and complex situations, ongoing education in ethics is fundamental. Participating in continuous ethical training keeps you sharp and attuned to the emerging issues within the field. It also enhances your ability to apply ethical principles to novel situations in practical and culturally competent ways.

In the digital age, issues of confidentiality extend to electronic communications and records. Staying informed about the latest in digital ethics and ensuring that you adhere to best practices in electronic record-keeping and communication is part of your ethical responsibility.

Lastly, remember that navigating ethical dilemmas is not a burden you must carry alone. Utilize the resources available to you —

professional organizations, ethics committees, and legal counsel when necessary. These resources can provide you with guidance and reinforce your actions when faced with ethical decisions.

As the mental health field progresses, so does the complexity of ethical decision-making. However, with a strong ethical foundation, a tactical approach grounded in empathy and respect, and the support of your peers and community, these challenges can be navigated successfully. The journey is an ongoing one, but each step you take strengthens not just your skills as a mental health technician, but also the integrity of the field itself.

Chapter 10:
Career Advancement and Opportunities

As you've garnered core competencies and cultivated resilience through your journey in mental health care, envisioning your professional trajectory becomes paramount. In Chapter 10, we delve into the manifold avenues for career progression, emphasizing the significance of networking and continuous professional development. To thrive, one must actively seek opportunities—immerse in varied environments, engage with diverse populations, and stay abreast of novel approaches in the field. Furthermore, we explore the transition into leadership roles, underscoring the skills necessary to mentor colleagues and effectively manage therapeutic teams. This chapter isn't just about climbing the professional ladder; it's about harnessing your potential, impacting lives profoundly, and leaving an indelible mark on the world of mental health. Here, you'll find the inspiration to stretch beyond your current role, to a future reflecting your dedication and passion.

Networking and Professional Development

As you venture into the field of mental health as a technician, it's not just about having technical know-how or clinical acumen; it's also about embracing the art of networking and the power of professional development. Networking is the invisible thread that connects opportunities, ideas, and careers. It's the conduit through which relationships are formed and nurtured, and through which you can find mentors, peers, and future job prospects. Professional development, on the other hand, refers to ongoing learning, training, and acquiring new skills that keep you current and relevant in the ever-evolving landscape of mental health care.

In this demanding field, staying connected and continuously learning are not merely optional; they are fundamental to personal and professional growth. Networking can be as simple as joining professional organizations related to mental health, attending conferences and workshops, or engaging in online forums and social media groups. Through these channels, you'll gain invaluable insights into the latest trends and research, and establish connections with like-minded professionals who share your passion and dedication.

The journey of professional development is deeply enriching. Continual learning not only broadens your knowledge base but also ignites a spark of enthusiasm for innovation in your practice. Whether it's attending webinars, participating in advanced training modules, or pursuing higher education, these pursuits enhance your qualifications and expertise, thus paving the way for career advancements.

Remember, as a mental health technician, you are part of a formidable community. You're not just doing a job; you're contributing to something that's much bigger than yourself—the mental well-being of society. Being actively involved in professional networks gives you a sense of collective mission and shared purpose. Attend association meetings or local community events where you can advocate for mental health and represent the essential role of technicians in the broader healthcare system.

Professional development can also involve obtaining additional certifications that open doors to further opportunities. The credentials you accumulate throughout your career are tangible evidence of your dedication and skill—a message to employers and clients alike that you are committed to excellence in your field. Certifications can also give you an edge, offering specialized training that could lead to more niche roles within mental health care.

The practical side of networking involves knowing how to present yourself. Create a solid, professional online presence. LinkedIn and professional portfolio websites are excellent platforms to showcase your qualifications, experiences, and aspirations. Your online profile is often the first impression you make; ensure it is a reflection of your professionalism and commitment to the field of mental health.

Mentorship is another key component of both networking and professional development. Seek out mentors who can offer guidance, advice, and support as you navigate your career path. In turn, as you gain experience, offering mentorship to others can be incredibly rewarding and beneficial to your own growth. Mentoring reinforces your knowledge, encourages leadership skills, and strengthens the profession as a whole by fostering a culture of education and mutual support.

While networking might appear daunting to some, approaching it with authenticity and curiosity can break down barriers. Engage in genuine conversations, ask insightful questions, and listen intently. Remember, every person you meet has the potential to teach you something valuable, whether it's a new perspective on practice, career advice, or even becoming a sounding board for your ideas.

It's also vital to remember that professional development is not a race; it's a continuous journey that aligns with your personal and professional goals. Set realistic, achievable goals for learning new skills or earning certifications and approach them with a disciplined, yet patient perspective. It's the steady accumulation of knowledge and connections that will fortify your career over time.

To sustain your networking and professional development efforts, keep an open mind. The field of mental health is dynamic, with new treatment modalities and technologies constantly emerging. Be willing to explore new avenues and stay adaptable—what works today may evolve tomorrow. Moreover, embrace changes with a proactive mindset that seeks not just to adjust but to lead and innovate.

Document and reflect on your professional development milestones. Keeping a record of your accomplishments, workshops attended, certificates earned, and conferences you've participated in can serve as a powerful reminder of your growth. This documentation will not only inspire you but will also be a persuasive element of your resume or portfolio.

Lastly, integrating your networking and professional development activities can lead to cultivating a balanced work-life. Your career should never come at the expense of your personal well-being. Ensure you strike a balance that allows you to be productive, happy, and healthy both in and out of the workplace.

Embark on this remarkable journey with a fervent mindset, utilizing every opportunity to network and grow professionally. Keep in mind that the true essence of mental health work lies in continuous learning and connecting—not just for the betterment of your career, but for the collective progress of mental health care provision. By investing in networking and professional development, you not only enrich your own career, but also contribute to the evolution of the entire mental health technician field.

In conclusion, networking and professional development are not destinations but transformative processes that equip you with the tools, knowledge, and connections to excel and flourish as a mental health technician. Let your passion fuel your growth, and allow your experiences to shape your career into a journey of lifelong learning and meaningful connections.

Exploring Different Settings and Populations

Pivoting within the comprehensive role of a Mental Health Technician (MHT), it's crucial to recognize the diverse settings and populations that one may encounter. This exploration is not just about understanding different working environments; it's about embracing the unique challenges and rewards that each setting offers. As MHTs, the adaptability to shift from one situation to another while maintaining a patient-centered approach is what sets apart a promising career from a truly impactful one.

Mental health care is not a monolith; it manifests in various forms across an array of settings, ranging from acute psychiatric units in hospitals to community-based group homes. Each setting not only demands a specialized skill set but also calls for an open mind and a compassionate heart. In hospitals, MHTs are often faced with high-intensity environments where quick thinking and rapid response to crises are daily occurrences. Here, the population comprises individuals in acute distress, requiring stabilization and intensive treatment.

On the other hand, residential treatment facilities offer a more long-term approach to care. MHTs in these settings work with clients who need ongoing support, often due to chronic mental illnesses or prolonged rehabilitation processes. The population here becomes akin to an extended family, with the overarching goal being progress and the cultivation of life skills within a therapeutic milieu.

Community mental health centers represent a different facet of mental health care, focusing on outpatient services and preventive care. MHTs engage with a broad demographic, from children to the elderly, each with distinct needs and stories. The work here leans towards continuity of care and community reintegration, necessitating an MHT's proficiency in case management and therapeutic interventions fitting for all ages.

Schools and educational settings also seek the expertise of MHTs, where they play a pivotal role in identifying and supporting students with behavioral or emotional challenges. Working collaboratively with educators and parents, MHTs are at the forefront of developing strategies that promote mental well-being and academic success. In these environments, sensitivity to developmental stages and an unwavering commitment to advocacy are essential.

Correctional facilities present a unique challenge for MHTs, coupling mental health services with the justice system. Here, the focus is on addressing the mental health issues of the incarcerated population, which are often complex and compounded by the stress of confinement. MHTs serve not only as caregivers but also as beacons of hope in a setting often devoid of it.

Each population within these settings has its nuances. For instance, working with veterans struggling with PTSD in a VA hospital will require an understanding of military culture and the traumas associated with combat. Similarly, providing care for individuals facing substance abuse in a rehab center demands knowledge of addiction and recovery processes.

Ambulatory care settings and day programs permit another flavor of mental health service provision. Here, MHTs support individuals who have sufficient stability to live independently but still benefit from structured therapeutic activities and socialization during the day. Flexibility and creativity in program planning become key qualities for MHTs in such environments.

Geriatric care adds an extra layer of sensitivity to the role of an MHT. Working with the elderly, especially those with dementia or age-related psychiatric conditions, calls for a gentle touch and patience. Knowledge of the aging process and empathy for the challenges it brings is paramount in these settings.

The foray into the mental health field is an invitation to endless growth, not only professionally but personally. Serving various populations, MHTs build a repertoire of experiences that hone their expertise and deepen their capacity for empathy. It's not just about changing lives; it's about being changed by the lives you touch.

Undoubtedly, working across different populations will expose MHTs to the wide spectrum of human experiences. Engaging with pediatric patients who are grappling with mental health issues at an early age is a complex task that requires not only clinical skills but also an inherent warmth and ability to connect with young minds.

Exploring these settings and populations is more than a journey through the landscape of mental health care; it's a quest for personal and professional fulfillment. As an MHT, you become the vanguard of wellness, an embodiment of strength and tenacity for those in your charge.

It also entails recognizing when to draw upon the collective wisdom of the interdisciplinary team. An MHT's ability to learn from psychologists, psychiatrists, social workers, and nurses enriches their understanding of each patient's journey, shaping a more holistic approach to care.

What sets the mental health field apart is the profound intersectionality of human life it presents. Cultivating cultural competence and understanding the socio-economic factors affecting mental health are not just professional responsibilities; they are moral imperatives for an MHT.

The MHT's path is not merely about career advancement; it's about embarking on a vocation that echoes with purpose and human connection. As you explore different settings and populations, you'll find that each new encounter expands your worldview, adding another layer to your professional tapestry. The dynamism of this field is the heartbeat that drives passionate individuals towards making a lasting difference.

Ultimately, as you explore the distinct settings and populations that will shape your career as a Mental Health Technician, remember that you're not just stepping into a job. You're stepping into countless stories, each waiting for you to play a pivotal role. In this vast mosaic of mental health care, your passion, skills, and dedication will light the way to a fulfilling and impactful career that transcends the personal triumph of success—it embodies the triumph of human spirit itself.

Leadership and Supervisory Roles

Within the realm of mental health care, these roles are pivotal not only for the seamless functioning of healthcare facilities but also for the growth and development of the mental health technicians themselves. Being a leader or a supervisor in this field isn't just about delegating tasks or managing a team; it's about influencing change, fostering a therapeutic environment, and guiding mental health technicians toward providing exemplary care.

Those who aspire to leadership roles must understand that it's not merely a job title but a commitment to excellence and a willingness to adopt a mindset of continuous improvement. Leadership in mental health care involves empathy, strong decision-making skills, and most importantly, the ability to inspire and motivate others. Supervisors must not only oversee the work of their team but also ensure the provision of compassionate and effective care to those in need.

As a leader in this field, one's responsibilities broaden from individual patient care to strategic oversight. It involves navigating the complexities of mental healthcare systems, maintaining high standards of practice, and fostering an environment that supports the holistic growth of both staff and patients. The role is dynamic and requires a balance of skills that extend beyond clinical expertise to managerial acumen.

Stepping into a supervisory role means being prepared to mentor new technicians, offering guidance based on experience and knowledge. It's about being a source of wisdom and support while also navigating the administrative aspects of care. Developing a sense of trust and respect with the team is essential, as is the ability to communicate effectively and manage conflicts should they arise.

Those in leadership positions must also navigate the challenges that come with a diverse team. They must be adept at cultural competence, understanding, and valuing the differences that each member brings to the table. In doing so, they enrich the therapeutic environment and ensure that care is inclusive and respectful of all backgrounds.

Leadership in mental health care is not about power, but about the power to empower. It involves recognizing and cultivating the potential in each team member, encouraging ongoing education, and supporting their professional growth. By investing in the development of your team, you are effectively strengthening the very fabric of mental health care.

It's critical to understand the dual nature of leadership roles in mental health, which involves balancing administrative duties with patient care responsibilities. This might include navigating the bureaucratic channels of healthcare administration while ensuring that the quality of care delivered is uncompromised.

Effective leaders in mental health care also play a crucial role in policy development and implementation within their settings. They must be both informed and opinionated on matters that affect mental health practice and advocate for policies that promote patient welfare and professional practice.

One must also acknowledge the role of technology in advancing mental health care and be prepared to lead teams through transitions and adaptations to new tools and treatments. Supervisors guide their teams in embracing change, overcoming the fear of the unknown, and utilizing technology to enhance patient care.

Feedback and evaluation are key components of supervisory roles. Leaders must be adept at providing constructive feedback that fosters growth while also being receptive to feedback regarding their own performance. The goal is to create a culture of open communication and mutual respect where feedback is seen as an opportunity for improvement.

Leadership involves a significant amount of responsibility, including legal and ethical decision-making. Supervisors in mental health care must ensure that the actions of their team adhere to the highest ethical standards and are in compliance with legal requirements. This protects the rights and interests of both patients and staff.

For a mental health technician stepping into a leadership role, it's crucial to embrace the responsibility of crisis management. Leaders are often the ones who must respond quickly and effectively to high-stress situations, making decisions that could significantly affect the well-being of both patients and staff.

Finally, being a leader in mental health care means championing for the mental well-being of your team. It involves recognizing the signs of burnout and fostering an atmosphere that prioritizes self-care and resilience. As a supervisor, your actions and attitude towards self-care can significantly influence your team's approach to their own well-being.

Leadership and supervisory roles in mental health require a unique blend of compassion, strength, foresight, and resilience. These roles are not static; they evolve with the landscape of mental health care and demand ongoing personal and professional development. For those called to leadership, it is both a profound responsibility and a meaningful opportunity to contribute to the fabric of a caring and effective mental health system.

Those seeking to rise into leadership positions must therefore be prepared to be a beacon of guidance, a pillar of strength, and a catalyst for change—striving to elevate not just themselves, but the entire milieu of mental health care provision. This journey is not for the faint of heart, but for those ready to embrace its challenges, it promises a fulfilling path where the impact on human lives is both tangible and deeply rewarding.

Chapter 11:
Self-Care for Mental Health Technicians

In the demanding world of mental healthcare, those who serve as custodians of others' psychological well-being must not overlook their own. It's crucial to remember that self-care is not merely a luxury but a cornerstone of professional longevity and effectiveness. As a mental health technician, you're often at the front line, absorbing the emotional and psychological shocks that are part and parcel of the healing process. Hence, embedding stress management techniques into your daily routine isn't just beneficial; it's essential. Develop a personal self-care regimen that resonates with your needs: whether that's through meditation, exercise, or creative pursuits, let it be the balm that restores your spirit. Don't underestimate the value of camaraderie in this field, either. Lean on your peers for support, for in the shared experiences, you'll find strength and validation. Cultivating resilience isn't simply about insulating yourself from the pressures of work—it's about transforming them into opportunities for growth.

Managing Stress and Avoiding Burnout

As we've explored the diverse responsibilities and the critical role of mental health technicians, it's important to recognize that the compassion and care you bring to every interaction doesn't come without its challenges. The demands of the job are not only physical but also profoundly emotional and psychological. In this sub-section, we'll delve into strategies for managing stress and avoiding burnout, essential practices that sustain you as a professional and a person.

Burnout can be a stealthy foe, particularly in a field rooted in empathy and service. You may not notice it creeping up until it begins to cast a shadow over both your work and personal life. It's characterized by feelings of exhaustion, cynicism, and a sense of reduced professional efficacy. To combat burnout, it's essential to develop a toolkit of stress management techniques tailored to your unique needs and work environment.

First and foremost, recognize the signs of stress in your body and mind. Do you feel a tightness in your chest, or is your mind constantly racing, even during downtimes? Acknowledge these signals without judgment and view them as indicators that it's time to activate your stress-response plan. This may include activities such as deep breathing exercises, brief meditative breaks, or engaging in physical activities that help release tension.

Effective time management is also key. Prioritize tasks and understand that it's okay to pause and reevaluate your to-do list. The ability to distinguish between urgent and important tasks can prevent the overwhelming feeling that everything must be done immediately and to perfection. Embrace the power of saying "no" or "not right now" when your workload becomes too onerous.

Building a robust support network is equally important. Colleagues may share similar experiences and can offer empathy and advice. Remember, it's a sign of strength to ask for help when you need it, whether it's delegating tasks when possible or seeking guidance on handling a challenging situation.

Maintaining a healthy work-life balance is vital. Your job is important, but it's just one aspect of your life. Make time for hobbies, relaxation, and social connections outside of work. These activities recharge your batteries and provide a healthy perspective that enriches both your personal and professional lives.

Don't underestimate the significance of a healthy lifestyle in stress management. Regular exercise, proper nutrition, and sufficient sleep are foundational pillars that affect your mental and emotional resilience. Consider them not as optional but as part of your job—it's self-care in its most basic form.

Professional development can play an unexpected role in managing stress. Enhancing your knowledge and skills can boost your confidence in dealing with difficult situations, reducing anxiety and stress. Whether through formal education or informal learning, staying current in your field can empower you and alleviate feelings of helplessness that often contribute to stress.

In moments of stress, it's crucial to practice mindfulness—staying grounded in the present rather than worrying about future tasks or ruminating on past events. Mindfulness can improve your response to stress and enhance your focus, allowing you to provide the best care possible while maintaining your calm.

Regular self-assessment is a proactive measure to monitor your stress levels and burnout risk. Reflecting on your job satisfaction, work environment, and even your physical and emotional well-being can provide insights into changes you might need to make to your professional approach or lifestyle.

Sometimes, despite all efforts, burnout can still take hold. If your strategies aren't enough, don't hesitate to seek professional assistance. Mental health practitioners can benefit as much from therapy as their patients do. It provides a confidential space to work through challenges and develop coping strategies, allowing you to return to your work rejuvenated.

Resilience-building is another tool for your stress-management arsenal. Resilience isn't about never facing difficulties; it's about bouncing back from challenges stronger than before. Developing resilience can involve setting personal goals, cultivating a positive outlook, and viewing challenges as opportunities for growth.

Give yourself permission to take breaks—real breaks. Step away from your work environment during your time off. An afternoon in nature, a day trip, or simply a tech-free day can provide a restorative break from the high demands of your role as a mental health technician.

Lastly, remember the "big picture." Remind yourself why you chose this profession. The work you do makes a profound difference in the lives of your patients. Connecting with this sense of purpose can reignite your passion and provide the inner strength to overcome stress and prevent burnout.

By integrating these stress management and burnout prevention strategies into your daily routine, you create a sustainable career that not only supports the well-being of your patients but also ensures your own longevity and satisfaction in this deeply rewarding field. Emotional resilience isn't just about surviving; it's about thriving, and as a mental health technician, you owe it to yourself and those you serve to nurture it.

With these tools at your disposal, and a commitment to self-care and professional growth, you're not merely well on your way to a successful career in mental health care—you're setting the stage for a fulfilling journey that honors both your personal well-being and your dedication to enhancing the lives of others.

Developing a Personal Self-Care Plan

This plan is not just an indulgence, it's a crucial part of being an effective mental health technician. The demands of the job require that you maintain your own wellness in order to provide the best care for others. Establishing a personal self-care plan can leave you feeling rejuvenated, ensuring you're ready to meet the challenges of each new day with resilience and compassion.

Firstly, personal self-care encompasses a variety of areas, some of which include physical health, mental well-being, emotional balance, and professional development. As you progress in your career, each of these areas can be nurtured to contribute to a rounded and robust personal health strategy.

Your physical well-being is foundational. Regular exercise not only keeps you fit but also releases endorphins that combat stress. Whether it's a daily walk, a yoga session, or a vigorous workout, finding physical activities that you enjoy is essential. Equally important is nutrition; the food you consume directly impacts your energy levels and mood. Crafting a balanced diet that fuels your body will empower you to handle demanding workloads.

Let's shift our focus onto mental well-being. As a mental health technician, you're no stranger to the impact of mental strain. Implementing strategies like mindfulness, meditation, or simply finding time to indulge in hobbies outside of work can provide a necessary reprieve from the rigors of your profession.

Emotional health is interlinked with mental well-being. Building emotional intelligence allows you to navigate your own feelings as well as those of others with finesse. Techniques such as journaling or engaging in reflective practices can enhance self-awareness and emotional regulation – skills that are invaluable both in your personal life and professional sphere.

Professional development is also an often-overlooked component of self-care. Pursuing continued education, attending workshops or conferences keeps you engaged and stimulates intellectual growth. This not only improves your job performance but also contributes to a sense of achievement and self-efficacy.

Sleep – the unsung hero of self-care. Adequate, restful sleep is non-negotiable. It's the time when your body repairs itself and your brain consolidates memories and learning from the day. Creating a sleep routine that aligns with your body's natural rhythms can greatly enhance your overall well-being.

Social connections play an integral role in a comprehensive self-care regimen. Building and maintaining positive relationships with colleagues, friends, and family provides a support network that bolsters you through tough times. Don't underestimate the healing power of laughter, love, and camaraderie.

Self-care also involves recognizing when you need help. There's strength in acknowledging that you can't handle everything alone and seeking assistance from a mentor, counselor, or support group is a proactive step. It demonstrates a commitment to maintain your mental health for your benefit and the benefit of those you care for.

Boundaries are also critical for self-preservation. Learning how to say 'no' or delegating tasks when appropriate protects your energy levels and prevents burnout. It's essential to identify your limits and communicate them effectively to others.

Moreover, a self-care plan must be dynamic, adapting as your personal and professional needs evolve. What works for you now might need adjustment later, and it's important to be attentive to those changing requirements.

Regular self-assessment is a valuable tool in the maintenance of your self-care plan. Periodically take stock of your physical, emotional, and mental states to identify areas needing attention or adjustment. This reflective practice ensures your self-care routine evolves in step with your life's ebbs and flows.

Also, don't overlook the importance of a conducive work environment. Personalize your workspace, where possible, to make it a calming and pleasant area. This can have a profound impact on your mood and productivity, making your job more enjoyable and sustainable.

Lastly, integrating your self-care plan into your daily life requires commitment. It's tempting to let self-care slide when work gets busy, but this is precisely when it's most needed. Prioritizing self-care is an investment in your capacity to deliver quality care to those in need.

Remember, your self-care plan is for you, designed by you. Tailor it to fit your life and make it something you look forward to. Small, consistent actions can have a powerful cumulative effect. Over time, these habits will become a natural part of your routine, leading to a more balanced, fulfilling career as a mental health technician.

To conclude, a personal self-care plan isn't just a luxury; it's an essential element of your toolkit as a mental health professional. It enables you to maintain your health and vitality, so you can bring your best self to your work and the patients who depend on you. Take the time to craft a self-care plan that resonates with you – your future self will thank you for it.

The Importance of Peer Support

As we've navigated the various facets of the mental health technician's role, one component persistently emerges as a vital pillar in the structure of mental well-being for professionals – peer support. The significance of peer support cannot be overemphasized; it envelopes the essence of shared experiences, empathetic listening, and mutual encouragement that bind mental health workers together in their challenging field.

No one truly walks alone in the journey of mental health care. Like the interlaced fingers of two hands, peer support represents the strength and interconnectedness essential for those who endeavor to aid others. Working in mental health, technicians often encounter experiences that can resonate deeply, demanding an outlet and a circle of understanding that typically only colleagues can offer.

Peer support within the mental health technician community can take on many forms, but at its core, it involves offering a listening ear, exchanging advice, sharing coping strategies, or simply being present for one another during tumultuous periods. This support is not a luxury; it is a fundamental tool to maintain professional efficacy and personal well-being.

Humans are inherently social creatures, and being able to relate one's experiences to others who can empathize provides a cathartic release from the mental loads carried. When mental health technicians share their stories and challenges with colleagues, they do more than express concerns—they partake in a collaborative effort to dissect, understand, and address the intricacies of their profession.

This collaborative effort leads to collective wisdom. Each individual's unique experiences, when shared, become a repository of knowledge that peers can draw from. New technicians can learn from those who have faced similar situations, while seasoned technicians can offer insights honed by years of practice. This synergy not only furthers individual knowledge but also fortifies the entire team against potential adverse events.

Moreover, there's a profound sense of camaraderie that arises from peer support groups. Knowing that there are others who have tackled similar challenges, who've experienced similar frustrations or jubilations, fosters a sense of belonging and community within the workforce that propagates morale.

Peer support also contributes significantly to the reduction of stigma surrounding mental health issues within the profession itself. By normalizing discussions about stress, burnout, and mental health challenges, these conversations pave the way for more open, honest, and beneficial interactions amongst colleagues.

It is crucial for mental health technicians to recognize the signs of stress and burnout in themselves and their peers. Through peer support, technicians can vigilantly monitor each other for such signs, offering interventions and encouraging professional help when necessary. Early recognition and action can prevent more severe consequences, allowing for continuous delivery of quality care to those who need it most.

Peer support contributes to creating a culture of learning and continuous improvement. Discussing cases, exchanging feedback, and brainstorming solutions to problems are opportunities for skill enhancement. This shared learning environment propels the growth of each technician, enriching their capacity to serve.

Implementation of structured peer support programs can further formalize these benefits. Such programs offer regular meetings, mentorship opportunities, and channels for anonymous sharing, which can be particularly beneficial for individuals who are less inclined to share openly.

Additionally, peer support is synonymous with resilience. As one faces the rigors of the mental health field, the shared strength that comes from a supportive network acts as a cushion against the potential impact of emotional stress. This resilience is not merely about surviving; it's about thriving and growing through adversity.

Peer support also ties into ethics and professional conduct. By engaging in discussions with peers, mental health technicians hold each other accountable, ensuring that the quality of care and adherence to ethical standards remain high. This mutual accountability safeguards the integrity of the profession and the well-being of the patients served.

For mental health technicians to fully engage in peer support, communication is key. Open lines of dialogue, whether through formal meetings, casual conversations, or digital platforms, ensure that peer support is readily accessible. Such communication channels must be nurtured and valued as central to the culture of mental health care.

Ultimately, the importance of peer support in the lives of mental health technicians is profound. Not only does it promote personal wellness and professional growth, but it also enhances the quality of care provided to patients. It represents a shared journey—a pilgrimage of sorts—that mental health technicians embark upon together, each step made lighter by the presence of a colleague beside them.

In closing, consider peer support as one of the greatest assets in your arsenal as a mental health technician. Embrace it, contribute to it, and witness how it transforms your professional journey and the lives of those around you into a mosaic of collaborative growth, success, and fulfillment.

Chapter 12:
The Future of Mental Health Care

As we journey deeper into the 21st century, the landscape of mental health care is undergoing transformative change, marked by groundbreaking innovation and pivotal shifts in policy. In this chapter, we shine a light on the upcoming advancements in treatment methods and technologies poised to revolutionize the way mental health services are delivered. These developments not only promise to enhance the efficacy of interventions but also seek to dismantle the barriers to access, rendering care more inclusive and personalized. This is a horizon where mental health professionals, including technicians, are not just witnesses but active participants and shapers of a new dawn in mental health care. Embrace this future as an active advocate, a beacon of change, ensuring that the mental health movement's momentum propels forward, building upon a foundation rooted in compassion and driven by unwavering determination to uplift and transform lives.

Innovations in Treatment and Technology

As we voyage through the transformative landscape of mental health care, we can't help but be astounded by the breathtaking advancements in treatment and technology shaping the trajectory of this vital field. Mental Health Technicians are at the forefront, embracing new tools and methodologies that revolutionize patient care and enhance their own professional capabilities.

Imagine a world where virtual reality transcends the boundaries of the mind, enabling individuals to confront phobias and traumas in a controlled, yet convincingly real environment. This is not a figment of science fiction but an increasingly commonplace tool in therapy. As a future mental health technician, you will find that such immersive technologies offer new pathways for breaking down the barriers to mental wellness.

Moreover, let us consider the integration of artificial intelligence (AI) into mental health services. AI can assist in early diagnosis, personalized treatment plans, and even provide round-the-clock support through chatbots. As a technician, your role may evolve to include working alongside these intelligent systems, facilitating their introduction to patient care, and ensuring they are utilized effectively and ethically.

As the digital era forges ahead, telepsychiatry and teletherapy have become more than buzzwords – they are reshaping access to care. Distance and lack of local resources no longer need to be prohibitive, as our screens become windows to compassionate support and professional guidance. As a mental health technician, you will likely become adept at facilitating these virtual sessions, ensuring that even those in remote regions receive the quality care they deserve.

Wearable technology, once the domain of fitness enthusiasts, has found its niche in monitoring mental health as well. Devices that can track sleep patterns, heart rate variability, and even predict anxiety attacks serve as adjuncts to traditional therapy, offering real-time data that empowers patients and clinicians alike. Your ability to interpret and act on this information will be paramount in delivering proactive care.

Advancements are not limited to gadgets and software. On the pharmaceutical front, precision medicine is making headway, where genetic testing helps to tailor medication to the individual, minimizing trial and error and reducing adverse effects. The mental health technician's role in liaising between patients and prescribers as part of this personalized approach cannot be overstated.

Amidst all this burgeoning technology, the human element remains irreplaceable. As such, collaborative care models are gaining traction, integrating multiple disciplines and leveraging a team approach to ensure holistic treatment. You will find yourself co-piloting efforts alongside psychiatrists, psychologists, and social workers, where your insights and observations contribute to refined and comprehensive care strategies.

The concept of digital therapeutics – using technology to deliver evidence-based therapeutic interventions – is also rising to prominence. These can enhance traditional treatment methods and provide additional support, guidance, and track progress over time. Mental health technicians thus become the bridge between patients and the digital world, educating and assisting in the adoption of these applications.

Moving forward, electronic health records (EHR) will continue to play a critical role in mental health care. The proficiency and attention to detail you'll need to maintain these records are crucial for legal compliance and coordinated care. Further, the EHR systems themselves are gradually incorporating predictive analytics, potentially identifying at-risk individuals before a crisis emerges.

Complementary and alternative therapies have always woven through mental health care, and now we see innovation sparkle in this space as well. Techniques like biofeedback, mindfulness apps, and online support communities are becoming integrated into standard care, offering a diverse palette from which patients can paint their pathways to wellness.

Furthermore, technology has been a catalyst for patient empowerment, providing platforms where they can be active participants in their care. Health information technology enables better communication with healthcare providers and access to a wealth of educational resources. As a mental health technician, be prepared to guide patients in using these tools for better self-management and advocacy.

Advances in robotics are even entering therapeutic spaces, aiding in the treatment of children with autism and seniors with dementia. These robots can provide consistent interactions, promote social skills, and offer comfort. As a technician, you'll need to stay informed about these innovations to effectively integrate them into therapy plans, all the while ensuring they supplement the irreplaceable human touch.

Let's not forget the paramountcy of data security and privacy in healthcare. Innovations in encryption and cybersecurity are continuously evolving to protect sensitive patient information. Your vigilance and proficiency in these areas will ensure trust in the healthcare system and safeguard the privacy and dignity of those you serve.

In the coming years, predictive analytics and big data will further shape mental health care delivery. This technology holds the promise of identifying trends, preventing relapse, and tailoring interventions to community needs. As a technician, your role may involve working within these data systems, translating insights into actionable interventions alongside your interdisciplinary team.

To close, recognize that innovation in mental health care is not merely about adopting new gadgets or algorithms; it's about cultivating a mindset of continuous learning and adaptation. As you embark on or advance in your career as a mental health technician, keep a pulse on the future. Embrace innovation with both arms and integrate it wisely and warmly into your practice, knowing that each step forward is a step toward hope and healing for those you serve.

Policy Changes and Their Implications

In the ever-evolving field of healthcare, mental health has seen significant shifts in how care is managed and provided. As you explore the impactful role of a mental health technician, understanding these legislative and policy shifts is as critical as grasping the techniques of care itself. Policies are the backbone that shapes practice, impacting every aspect from funding to the day-to-day operations in a mental health facility. Let's delve into the recent policy changes and consider how these adjustments carry weighty implications for those working on the front lines of mental health care.

Policy reforms often respond to cultural and societal demands for improved mental health services. For instance, the past decade has seen an increase in the destigmatization of mental health, consequently leading to policies that push for better access to services. One such example is the enhancement of insurance coverage for mental health issues, paralleling that of physical health conditions. This inclusivity in insurance is a stride toward equality in healthcare, providing patients with more comprehensive coverage for their mental health treatment, which cascades into increased demand for skilled mental health technicians to meet this need. As a technician, you'll witness first-hand the increase in clients who can now receive necessary care due to these policy changes.

The implications of policy changes don't stop at the patient's level. Within the walls where care is administered, these policies lead to the creation of new roles and responsibilities for mental health technicians. For instance, the integration of behavioral health with primary care opens new avenues for professionals to work collaboratively, necessitating technicians to develop a broader understanding of overall patient health and care coordination competencies.

Moreover, privacy regulations, such as changes to the Health Insurance Portability and Accountability Act (HIPAA), have significant implications for mental health technicians. You must stay vigilant, remaining informed on policy updates and training requirements to ensure the confidentiality and ethical handling of patient information. Compliance with updated regulations is not only legal but also a matter of ethical responsibility to those entrusted to your care.

With the rise of telehealth services, particularly magnified by the COVID-19 pandemic, policies surrounding remote care have leaped forward. As a result, mental health technicians now find themselves at the junction of providing care that is both traditional and technologically driven. New policies have broadened the scope of telehealth, allowing more patients to access mental health services from the comfort of their homes. This paradigm shift includes understanding telehealth regulations, incorporating digital competencies into your skill set, and adapting your patient interaction techniques to a virtual setting.

Policy changes also throw into sharp relief the importance of continuous education and certification. As Medicaid and other insurance providers alter requirements for billing and reimbursement, staying updated with certifications becomes more than self-improvement; it becomes a necessity to maintain employment. Mental health technician training programs are thus tailored to meet these evolving standards, urging you to embrace a mindset of lifelong learning.

Furthermore, policies are steering toward a more holistic view of mental health care. Legislative initiatives that push for integrative care models mean mental health technicians must be well-versed in interdisciplinary approaches, working seamlessly with a team of healthcare providers. This means expanding your worldview to consider a variety of aspects of patient care, from physical comorbidities to socioeconomic factors influencing mental health.

In regard to crisis intervention, recent policy updates enforce more stringent procedures and training for handling psychiatric emergencies. For you, as a mental health technician, this calls for honing your skills in de-escalation techniques and emergency response—ensuring patient and staff safety during critical incidents.

Workplace safety policies have also seen updates, particularly in terms of worker protections. Mental health technicians often face challenging situations that can put them at risk of burnout or emotional fatigue. Updated policies may offer better support structures, such as mandated staff-to-patient ratios or required breaks, ensuring a safer and more supportive work environment. Understanding and advocating for these changes not only benefits you but also enhances patient care.

While polices shape the environment, they also highlight the importance of patient advocacy. Current health policy reforms often involve patient input and emphasize patient-centered care. These changes elevate the role of the mental health technician as an advocate, as you're in a prime position to voice the concerns and needs of the patients you work closely with.

Amidst these changes, the role of cultural competency has taken center stage. Policies that foster inclusive care for diverse populations mean that mental health technicians must educate themselves on cultural sensitivities and the specific needs of various demographic groups. The implications for practice are profound, as these policies drive the need for a more diverse and culturally literate workforce.

Lastly, as we contemplate policy changes and their implications for mental health technicians, it's crucial to consider your own development in leadership qualities. As these shifts occur, opportunities arise for mental health technicians to take on greater responsibilities, influencing policy through participation in professional organizations or community advocacy groups. Your growth in this field can be bolstered by an understanding of policy and an engagement with the community you serve.

At the heart of these policy changes lies a calling to remain adaptable, informed, and proactive. As mental health care continues to advance, these policies will inevitably alter the landscape of care provision. For you, an aspiring or current mental health technician, they represent opportunities to become a trailblazer in the field— embracing change, advocating for best practices, and contributing to a future where mental health care is accessible, equitable, and holistic. In the end, these policies are more than regulations; they are the stepping stones on your path to making a positive and lasting impact in the lives of those who seek mental wellness.

Advocacy and the Mental Health Movement

As we look ahead to the future of mental health care, one of the most influential factors shaping this landscape is the rise of advocacy and the burgeoning mental health movement. It's not just a peripheral activity; it has become a central tenet in the evolution and reformation of mental health services on a global scale. As you contemplate a career as a Mental Health Technician, understanding the interplay between advocacy and professional practice can be a beacon guiding you through the complexities of this field.

First and foremost, advocacy in mental health involves raising awareness about mental health issues, fighting stigma, educating the public, and lobbying for policy change. Mental health advocates are the vanguards who champion the rights and needs of those with mental illness. They push for better services, improved treatment options, and equitable access to mental health care for all individuals, irrespective of their socioeconomic status.

As a Mental Health Technician, immersing yourself in the advocacy realm is both empowering and enlightening. You have the opportunity to advocate for your patients on an individual level, ensuring their voices are heard within the care setting. Advocacy also means educating and empowering your patients to advocate for themselves, which is an integral component of their recovery and overall well-being.

The mental health movement is a diverse and dynamic force for change, composed of individuals and organizations committed to eradicating the barriers to quality mental health care. It encompasses a broad range of activities, from grassroots community work to international campaigns. Aspects of this movement involve tackling the stigma often associated with mental illness, promoting a more profound public understanding of mental health, and fostering a shift in societal attitudes.

Stigma is a formidable foe. It propagates misunderstanding and leads to discrimination. Advocates work tirelessly to dismantle the prejudices that can prevent individuals from seeking the help they need. As a professional in the mental health field, you'll be at the frontline of this battle, modeling acceptance and affirming the dignity of each individual you encounter.

The movement also focuses on legislative advocacy – a critical arena where policies and laws governing mental health care are shaped. Mental Health Technicians, coupled with their clinical insights, can play a pivotal role in informing and influencing policy. By sharing your on-the-ground experiences, you contribute valuable perspectives that can shape better mental health care policies and practices.

Educational advocacy is another sphere that plays a key role in mental health. This involves the provision of resources, training, and information to families, educators, and other stakeholders. As a technician, you might have the chance to engage in community outreach programs, workshops, or seminars that help to break down complex mental health concepts into understandable and actionable information.

With the ascension of digital platforms and social media, advocacy efforts have been supercharged. Campaigns can gain momentum faster than ever before, reaching a global audience and mobilizing people for action. This digital wave brings an opportunity for Mental Health Technicians to interact with larger networks, share their experiences, and raise consciousness around mental health matters.

Collaboration is at the heart of effective advocacy. Building alliances with other health care professionals, community leaders, and organizations enhances the collective impact. It's through these partnerships that systemic changes can be fostered. In this light, networking isn't just about professional development; it's about constructing a web of mutual support for significant change.

Advocacy also happens at the micro-level – within the walls of mental health facilities themselves. Advocating for quality improvement and patient-centered care practices is an area where Mental Health Technicians can have a direct influence. By understanding the power dynamics and governance structures, you can become an integral part of the transformations within your workplace that benefit both staff and patients alike.

Recovery-oriented care is an advocacy area that aligns closely with the values of the mental health movement. This approach emphasizes hope, empowerment, and the individual's own goals and strengths. As a Mental Health Technician, your role in promoting and applying a recovery-oriented framework can facilitate profoundly positive outcomes for individuals in your care.

The journey of advocacy is not without its challenges; it demands resilience, passion, and unswerving commitment. You will face obstacles and resistance. Yet, the importance of this endeavor can't be overstated. Advocacy affects the quality of care your patients will receive, the accessibility of mental health services, and ultimately, it can alter the landscape of mental health for future generations.

When you align with the mental health movement, you are doing more than just performing a job. You are part of a cause. You are a change agent in a world that desperately needs informed, compassionate, and proactive individuals in the realm of mental health. Your advocacy, no matter the scale, echoes far beyond the immediate horizons and can ignite sparks of hope and progress.

As you march forward in your career, let advocacy be the pulse of your professional ethos. Strengthen your resolve to serve not just as a technician, but as an advocate for those who might not have the strength to advocate for themselves. View every interaction, every learning opportunity, and every challenge as a chance to further the noble cause of the mental health movement.

In this spirit of change, remember that your path as a Mental Health Technician isn't just about the skills you acquire or the knowledge you amass – it's about embodying a philosophy that respects, nurtures, and elevates the mental health of everyone. You are an essential thread in the fabric of a society striving for wellness, and your every action can contribute to the grand tapestry of mental health advocacy.

Conclusion

As we reach the final pages of our exploration into the dynamic and ever-evolving field of mental health technicians, we must pause to reflect on the journey we've embarked upon throughout this book. The landscape of mental health care is vast and complex, yet at its core, it is about human connection, empathy, and the relentless pursuit of wellness and understanding.

From understanding the intricacies of mental health and defining the role of the mental health technician in Chapter 1, to discussing the growing demand for these essential professionals in our communities in Chapter 2, we've unraveled layers of this meaningful occupation. This role is not just a job; it's a call to service—one that requires a special blend of skills, patience, and compassion that has been meticulously outlined in Chapter 3.

Chapter 4 illuminated the pathways forged for aspiring mental health technicians, shedding light on the importance of education and certification. The attainable steps outlined are your stepping stones to making a palpable difference in the lives of those grappling with mental health challenges.

Providing an intimate glance into a day in the life of a mental health technician, Chapter 5 offered a vivid image of the daily responsibilities and ethical obligations that accompany this line of work. These responsibilities underscore the weight and impact of every action within the therapeutic environment, a theme further enhanced in Chapters 7 and 8.

The diverse patient population depicted in Chapter 6 should serve as a reminder that every person who walks through the doors of a mental health facility brings with them a tapestry of experiences and needs. Our ability to offer culturally sensitive, personalized care is what builds trust and fosters successful outcomes.

Understanding crisis intervention and maintaining safety, as we have seen in Chapter 7, are critical components of the job. They require a balance of firmness and gentleness, an ability to be a steadfast presence amidst chaos and uncertainty.

Furthermore, the therapeutic environment is not merely a backdrop but is an active and influential character in the treatment journey, as Chapter 8 so thoroughly conveyed. The harmonized symphony of therapeutic modalities and the right environment triggers a healing response, a concept that all mental health technicians should embrace wholeheartedly.

The pillars of legal and ethical considerations, detailed in Chapter 9, should be etched into the consciousness of every mental health professional. Upholding these principles is not just about adhering to the law but about fortifying the bond of trust so essential between the technician and their patients.

With Chapter 10's forward-looking perspective on career advancement, the possibilities for growth should inspire you to aim high and dream big. Your career trajectory is not set in stone; it's fluid, filled with numerous opportunities for those who seek them with vigor and determination.

Chapter 11 brought into focus the importance of self-care, an aspect of this profession that cannot be overstated. Cultivating resilience, identifying stressors, and developing personal self-care plans ensures longevity and fulfillment in your career, which in turn enhances the quality of care you provide.

Lastly, Chapter 12 should serve as a beacon of progress, highlighting the advancements in mental health care that are on the horizon. Advocacy, policy changes, and innovations are reshaping the future—the future you will be a part of molding and influencing as a mental health technician.

In conclusion, this book is not merely a guide but a companion on your transformative journey. The mental health field awaits with its challenges and triumphs, its moments of deep sadness and profound joy. The field of mental healthcare needs tenacious, compassionate individuals who are not simply looking for a career but are looking to make a difference in the world—one life at a time.

May this book serve as your north star, illuminating the path towards a fulfilling professional life in mental health care. As you continue to grow, learn, and evolve, remember that your role is vital, your impact immeasurable, and your potential boundless. The world of mental health is richer for your contribution. May you embark upon this journey with courage, wisdom, and an unwavering commitment to those you serve.

Appendix A:
Resources for Mental Health Technicians

The journey you're embarking upon as a Mental Health Technician is both substantial and profoundly rewarding. You are joining a community of compassionate and skilled individuals dedicated to making a difference in the lives of those who navigate mental health challenges. Beyond the foundational knowledge and insights you've garnered through our earlier chapters, this appendix is dedicated to equipping you with an arsenal of resources to support and enhance your career.

Professional Organizations and Associations

The American Association of Psychiatric Technicians (AAPT)

A professional organization dedicated to the support and advancement of psychiatric technicians. Membership can offer networking opportunities, information on best practices, and continuing education resources.

The National Association of Mental Illness (NAMI)

An advocacy group offering educational programs and support for mental health professionals. They provide resources for further learning and community engagement.

The National Federation of Families for Children's Mental Health

A national family-run organization focused on the issues of children and youth with emotional, behavioral, or mental health needs and their families.

Educational Resources

Substance Abuse and Mental Health Services Administration (SAMHSA)

Offers comprehensive information and training on various mental health topics, including substance abuse and recovery.

Mental Health America (MHA)

Provides educational materials and toolkits for mental health professionals to enhance their knowledge and capacity to assist those in need.

Psychiatric-Mental Health Nurse (PMH)

Provides a variety of online courses and webinars for continued professional development in psychiatric-mental health.

Online Journals and Publications

The Journal of Mental Health

An international forum for the latest research in the mental health field.

Psychiatric Services

A journal providing research and commentary on the delivery of behavioral health services.

Networking Opportunities

Networking can be a powerful tool in your career progression. Consider attending national conferences, regional workshops, and local seminars to connect with peers, mentors, and leaders in the mental health field.

Continuing Education and Workshops

Check for available workshops and seminars offered by universities and colleges, or even online platforms that specialize in mental health education. Look for accredited programs that can provide professional development credits.

Online Forums and Support Groups

Engage with online communities, such as **Psychiatric Technician Forums** or **LinkedIn Groups**, to find support, share experiences, and discuss the latest trends and challenges in the field.

As you forge ahead, remember that the wellspring of passion that drew you to this profession is the same force that will fuel your growth and effectiveness. Use these resources as stepping stones on your path to excellence. You have the potential to be influential in shaping the burgeoning field of mental health care, one life at a time. Embrace learning, seek connection, and above all, cultivate empathy and resilience within yourself. Your commitment is a beacon of hope, and your impact will extend far beyond what you can measure.

Glossary of Terms

Welcome to the Glossary of Terms, where clarity meets your curiosity. Each term listed here is a beam of light on the path to comprehending the multifaceted landscape of mental health care. From technical jargon to the soft skills that make up the fabric of this field, this collection of definitions is crafted to lift the veil on any uncertainties you might encounter as you dive deeper into the world of Mental Health Technicians. Let's illuminate these concepts together, paving the way for a future where terms are not barriers, but bridges to greater understanding.

A

- **Advocacy** - The act of speaking, writing, or acting in favor of a cause or individual, particularly within the context of mental health, to promote better care, policies, and understanding.

- **Assessment** - The process of gathering information about a patient's mental, emotional, and behavioral health to make informed decisions about their care.

B

- **Behavioral Health** - A term that encompasses the promotion of mental health, the prevention and treatment of mental and substance use disorders, and recovery support.

- **Burnout** - A state of emotional, physical, and mental exhaustion caused by prolonged stress and/or overworking, particularly in helping professions like mental health care.

C

- **Crisis Intervention** - Emergency psychological care provided to individuals experiencing a mental health crisis, aimed at de-escalating the situation and providing immediate support.

- **Cultural Sensitivity** - The awareness of and respect for the differences in beliefs, values, practices, and cultural factors that influence an individual's mental health and well-being.

D

- **De-escalation Techniques** - Strategies used to decrease the intensity of a conflict or potentially violent situation, often implemented by Mental Health Technicians to ensure safety and resolve crises.

E

- **Emotional Resilience** - The ability to adapt to and recover from stressful situations or crises, an essential trait for Mental Health Technicians to maintain personal well-being in challenging work environments.

- **Ethics** - Moral principles that govern a person's behavior or the conducting of an activity, critical for ensuring professional integrity and patient trust in mental health care.

I

- **Interpersonal Skills** - The ability to communicate and interact effectively with others, often used to build relationships with patients and collaborate with health care teams.

L

- **Licensure** - The process of being granted a license to practice as a Mental Health Technician, which may vary by region and typically involves meeting certain educational and training requirements.

M

- **Mental Health** - A state of well-being in which an individual realizes their own abilities, can cope with normal stresses of life, can work productively, and is able to contribute to their community.
- **Multidisciplinary Team** - A group composed of professionals from various specialties who work together to provide comprehensive care to individuals with complex health needs.

P

- **Patient Rights** - Legal and ethical entitlements related to medical privacy, informed consent, and participation in their own care, all upheld by Mental Health Technicians and other health care professionals.

R

- **Recovery Support** - Assistance and resources provided to individuals recovering from mental illness or addiction, aimed at helping them manage their condition and maintain their well-being.

S

- **Self-Care** - Practices and activities that an individual engages in on a regular basis to reduce stress and maintain and enhance short- and long-term health and well-being.

T

- **Therapeutic Modalities** - Varied treatments used to address mental health issues, which can include counseling, medication management, and alternative therapies.

We hope this Glossary of Terms serves as your trusty compass, providing clear direction through the terrain of your journey into the mental health field. With each term now defined, you're more than equipped with knowledge — you're empowered. May you utilize this profound understanding in manifesting your vision of support, compassion, and dedication as a future Mental Health Technician.

Appendix B:
Sample Templates and Checklists for Daily Use

As we navigate the intricate tapestry that is mental health care, every tool and resource at our disposal becomes a beacon of support for both technician and patient alike. The need for structure and consistency in daily tasks is a cornerstone of this noble profession. This appendix serves as a gateway to practical implements—sample templates and checklists—that you can adapt and employ within your own routines, making each day a measured stride towards excellence.

Daily Task Checklist

Whether it's a bustling morning or a quiet afternoon, a checklist can clarify your duties and help to reinforce a symbiotic rhythm with both colleagues and those you serve. Below is an example of what your daily checklist might include:

1. Review patient schedules and appointments

2. Check on medication inventories and flag any needs for re-orders

3. Prepare and organize patient records for the day's sessions

4. Conduct room and equipment safety checks

5. Coordinate with the multidisciplinary team for patient care plans

6. Set aside time for charting and documentation after each patient interaction

7. Review any patient communication that requires follow-up

Remember that these tasks are not merely boxes to tick off; they're threads in the larger fabric of a patient's journey to wellness. Approach each with the mindfulness they deserve.

Weekly Review Template

Amidst your weekly odyssey, pause to reflect on the progress and waves made. The Weekly Review Template can be your compass, guiding you through the accomplishments and learnings of the past week and setting the stage for the one ahead. Here's what that might look like:

- Summarize the week's major achievements
- Identify any challenges faced and solutions found
- Record any notable changes in patient progress
- Gather insights from team feedback and discussions
- Plan for upcoming events or changes in the routine
- Assess your own professional growth and areas for improvement

When you chronicle your week, it isn't just about accountability, but growth. The act of reviewing and planning is a ladder to mastery.

Patient Interaction Checklist

Each interaction with a patient is a delicate dance of compassion and professionalism. Here's a sample checklist to carry you gracefully through those essential moments:

1. Greet the patient warmly and with a reassuring presence
2. Review the patient's current care plan and any recent updates
3. Ensure you have all necessary materials ready for the session

4. Maintain a therapeutic environment throughout the interaction

5. Listen actively and provide interventions as identified in the care plan

6. Document the interaction accurately and promptly after its conclusion

7. Check in with the patient regarding their comfort level and any concerns before they leave

Each checkpoint is a commitment to nurturing trust and safety within the therapeutic relationship.

Monthly Inventory and Supplies Checklist

Stay ever-prepared by ensuring essential supplies are well-stocked and in working order. A Monthly Inventory and Supplies Checklist may include items such as:

1. Count and log medication stock levels

2. Check expiration dates on all consumable items

3. Audit first-aid and emergency equipment

4. Review and restock office supplies and stationery

5. Perform a thorough analysis of any frequently used tech or equipment

6. Ensure hygiene materials are sufficient for maintaining a clean environment

Maintaining inventory is not merely administrative—it's ensuring a seamless canvas on which the daily art of care is painted.

Let these samples guide you, but remember that they are canvases awaiting your personal touch. Customize them to the color and contour of your setting, and you'll forge a practice of not just proficiency, but of poetry.

May you use these tools not just as aids, but as launching pads for service that turns professionalism into a form of alchemy that transforms lives—including your own. Through this practical wisdom, you can find the rhythm that resonates with the pulse of your mission as a mental health technician.

Online Review Request for This Book

If this book has empowered you to take bold steps towards your future in mental health care, consider sharing your journey through a review online; your insights could light the path for others standing at the threshold of this rewarding career.